The New SLIMMING and HEALTH Workbook

The perfect balance of diet, exercise and natural food supplements, tailored to meet your own, unique needs and bringing with it the rewards of health, fitness and the ideal weight for you.

By the same author:
ABOUT LAETRILE
ACUPUNCTURE TREATMENT OF PAIN
AMINO ACIDS IN THERAPY
CANDIDA ALBICANS
INSTANT PAIN CONTROL
OSTEOPATHY
YOUR COMPLETE STRESS-PROOFING PROGRAMME

The New SLIMMING and HEALTH Workbook

Eat well — feel well — lose weight —
develop the action plan that's right for *you*

by

Leon Chaitow
N.D., D.O.

THORSONS PUBLISHING GROUP

First published in March 1985 as
Your Own Slimming and Health Programme.
First published in this new, revised and updated
format in 1989.

This edition revised and edited by Jane Bishop
Illustrated by Alex Ayliffe

© LEON CHAITOW 1989

*All rights reserved. No part of this book may be
reproduced or utilized in any form or by any means,
electronic or mechanical, including photocopying,
recording or by any information and retrieval system,
without permission in writing from the Publisher.*

British Library Cataloguing in Publication Data

Chaitow, Leon
  The new slimming and health workbook.
  1. Man. Health. Self-care 2. Physical
  fitness. Slimming
  I. Title
  613

ISBN 0-7225-1764-5

Published by Thorsons Publishers Limited,
Wellingborough, Northamptonshire NN8 2RQ,
England.

Printed in Great Britain by Richard Clay Limited,
Bungay, Suffolk
Typeset by MJL Limited, Hitchin, Hertfordshire

10 9 8 7 6 5 4 3 2 1

Contents

Chapter

1	Setting your target	9
2	How well do you eat?	17
3	Fitness and relaxation	35
4	What is your metabolic type?	47
5	Diet for your metabolic type	59
6	General dietary advice	73
7	Advanced exercises	79
8	Endocrine dysfunctions	97
9	Further nutritional needs	105
10	Putting it all together	119
	Index	127

I dedicate this book to Irene, Max Alkmini and Sasha, with love.

Setting your target

The task of achieving the ideal weight for each person is a personal matter. We are all possessed of unique characteristics, metabolically speaking, and therefore there is no single diet that is right for all people. In this book I have moved away from the normal, gimmicky, slimming diet, and I have also taken the position that without achieving a reasonable level of health and fitness, there is no way in which a correct body weight can be achieved.

Without an individual approach to our nutritional and exercise patterns, designed to meet our particular needs, there is small chance of achieving health or an optimum weight. The book that has resulted from these aims is, I believe, capable of nothing less dramatic than the complete restructuring of the health level of anyone who carries out its advice. Vital health, and your own ideal body weight, are the prizes. The effort is yours. Twenty-five years' experience in this field has convinced me of the validity of the programme.

It is presented in stages, to allow you to make the changes necessary to achieve these goals. There is no ideal weight for height, since a different genetic pattern is inborn in each of us. You cannot turn a bulldog-type into a whippet. You can, however, turn a bulldog into the healthiest and fittest of his particular type. That is our aim for all types of body shape and weight. All the slimming books on earth will not produce good health. *Good health, however, leads inevitably to the ideal weight.* Health comes first and the programme, if completed as designed, will provide the chance for achieving that goal. With that will come your ideal weight.

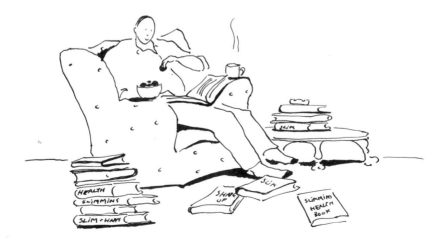

Optimum health

Once you have read this book you will have the opportunity to revolutionize your health status to a point where you can reach levels of vitality, and what has been termed 'high level wellness', undreamed of till now. You can do this by your own efforts if you follow, step by step, the programme which we will work out together as we progress through the book.

By identifying the individualized needs of your body, you will determine your dietary pattern, your exercise pattern, and other aspects of the programme.

The peak of health, and the ideal weight for your particular metabolic type, is your goal. Optimum health is a fantastic goal, for it means that you can start to realize your full potential as a human being. What a marvellous triumph that represents, and what opportunities for achieving other goals, which were previously out of reach because you were functioning at a lower level of health.

By taking the programme one step at a time, as it is designed, you are, by degrees, taking control of your life, and are learning to provide your body with all that it requires in terms of nutrition, exercise and stress reduction. Body and mind are catered for and, as you introduce changes to your present lifestyle, so you will know that you are accepting responsibility for yourself and for your health.

As this process continues, and as health benefits accrue, so your attitude towards yourself will alter. You will realize that many of your past problems are the direct result of your not having met the individual unique needs of your body and mind. If happiness in this world matters, then health certainly does, for one flows from the other, as does the ability to be of help to others.

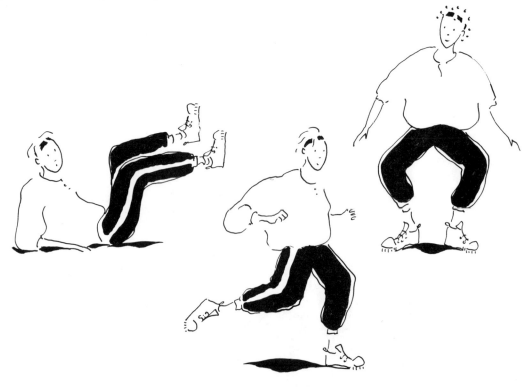

Series of tasks

The task of restructuring your whole eating and exercise pattern may appear very formidable indeed. It is, if you look at the final objective and then look at where you are starting from, and realize the gulf that lies between. On the other hand, if you see the objective, and the series of gentle stages in between, clearly signposted, then the journey seems less of a mammoth task. For the progression from where you are to where you are going is only a series of small tasks, each one made easier by the fact that you have accomplished previous ones, and are feeling the benefits.

The initial necessity for the success of the programme and the realization of its objectives is that you believe in the possibility of success, and that you understand what we are asking you to do, and why. The *why* of it all is important, because if the programme makes sense to you intellectually this will reinforce the emotional determination that you have to go for your target. *Please read the book through before starting the first stages of the programme.* You will then realize clearly that the various stages of the programme lead into one another, and complement each other. It is no good only dipping into aspects of the programme, though it would doubtless do some good, because the whole concept is designed to provide you with insights upon which you can then act, allowing you to take charge of your life, your health, and your ideal weight level.

There will be periods of depression or stress when you are tempted to throw it all in and binge as you may have done in the past but I will give you guidelines regarding what you can do in such an event, and we consider practical steps to counteract this all too common happening.

Whatever doubts you may have, it *is* possible to achieve enormous improvements in health, and to adjust to your own ideal weight by the methods described in the following chapters.

Know your type

Slimming diets come and slimming diets go, but the problems they aim to solve appear to go on forever. A simple and undeniable observation is that few of these diets, whether aimed at weight reduction or at health promotion, take into account one all important and irrefutable fact. We are all different. Individuality is not a vague theory; it is well established[1] that we all have different nutritional needs within a broadly similar framework. Unless we can identify and supply these individual needs we cannot achieve optimum health or, if that is the aim and the need, our ideal weight.

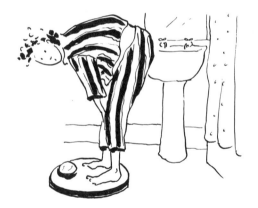

Aiming at weight reduction as a first and prime target is almost always a mistake. If you are unnaturally overweight then that fact is but a symptom of an imbalance, a dysfunction. This is what must be dealt with; the weight problem will then take care of itself. Without health there is no chance of maintaining a stable ideal weight.

[1] *Biochemical Individuality.* Roger Williams Ph.D., (University of Texas Press).

Short-term measures only achieve short-term results. If that is what you want then grab the first high-protein, low-fat, or high-fibre diet that is currently in vogue. The results will be problematical, for the diet you choose may or may not suit your real biological needs. Only by identifying your particular make-up, and then proceeding from that secure base, can you hope to ensure that what you eat is what you really need. In this way you can achieve your prime aim, which is to be healthy, and from this will flow the eradication of your particular weight problem.

The problem of being overweight may not even be a problem at all, for some people. By this I mean that, for some, it is normal and natural and genetically correct to be carrying more than the average weight. For others this is not so and the extra weight being carried is a real threat to health and longevity. The first step in deciding whether or not to try and lose weight therefore is to ascertain the likelihood of succeeding.

If you are genetically overweight there is little point in trying to alter your inborn characteristics, unless you have 'gilded the lily' and added to the weight bonus that nature handed you. If you are unnaturally overweight then we must look at that fact as we would any other symptom of bodily dysfunction (ill health). Remember always that it is a mistake to treat a symptom without dealing with its underlying cause. We are all biologically and biochemically unique. We are all different in our genetic and hormonal characteristics, and no one pattern of treatment or dietary regimen will suit all people. If we are to succeed in successfully adjusting your weight to what it ought to be, we have to identify what your particular pattern of biological individuality demands. The pattern of eating that makes you healthy will make you slim, if it is natural for you to be slim. Our aim is health with slimness as an added extra, which will derive from your body being given the nutritional pattern that it requires.

There are a variety of factors involved in assessing your particular biological type, a task which must be undertaken before deciding upon the actual programme. In order, however, to arrive at a reasonably accurate assessment of your individual needs nutritionally, we must have eliminated from the diet substances which, by their very nature, might confuse the picture and make assessment more difficult.

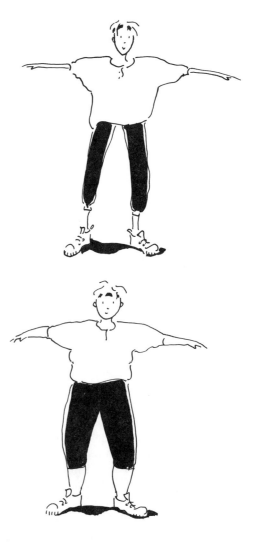

We need to assess, for example, thyroid function by means of a very simple series of early morning temperature recordings. If the diet contains substances such as caffeine (tea, coffee, chocolate, cola drinks, etc) during this phase of testing we may not get accurate and reliable results. If the diet contains sugar then we are also likely to have a confused picture. If you are prone to allergic or sensitivity reactions to particular foodstuffs then again our results may be confused. So we must start our quest for health and a balanced weight by eliminating harmful factors from the daily pattern of life.

The second stage is to identify your particular physiological make-up. Finally we must build into the dietary pattern individually indicated nutrient supplements. These might be minerals, vitamins, enzymes or amino acids which your particular profile indicates as being desirable. The dietary pattern indicated, together with supplements, should then be followed for a period during which time your health and well-being can be expected to improve tremendously.

While you are achieving your weight goal you will automatically be improving your overall physiological functioning. You will be getting healthier day by day, and the benefits in terms of energy, well-being, and the disappearance of a multitude of minor health problems, will be your reward for not attempting short-cuts to health.

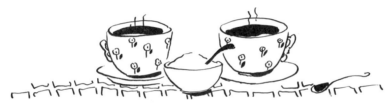

Health plan:

Stage 1   Elimination of undesirable factors.

Stage 2   Assessment of individual metabolic type.

Stage 3   Introduction of supplements and dietary pattern.

Concurrent with these three stages runs an extremely important exercise and relaxation programme which is designed to fit your individual needs and which will be discussed in the appropriate chapters.

This pattern has been followed by thousands of my patients over the past twenty five years and, where it has been correctly applied, the result in terms of health and well-being have often been spectacular. Weight has almost always adjusted itself towards its norm. Sometimes, when it was required, the same pattern of nutrition and exercise, tailored to the individual, has produced a weight increase. This has only happened where the patient's weight was below his optimum needs at the outset. So when we talk of optimum weight we are not talking about insurance charts of mythical 'ideal weights', but about *your particular needs* and *your healthy weight.*

Body mass

It is quite remarkable to realize that, for many years now, millions of people have been attempting to achieve a mythical ideal weight based on a wrong conception of what we should weigh. It has been demonstrated by one of the leading experts on the subject, Dr Ancel Keys, that the charts used by insurance companies are incorrect in their assumption of health risks attached to mild overweight states.

The ideal human weight (based on height for weight ratios) is 5 to 10lb (2.3 to 4.5 kilos) *too low* in insurance charts. He has shown that it is not relevant, as far as life expectancy is concerned, to be up to 20lb (9 kilos) above average weights. Above 20 lb (9 kilos) over average weight does, however, carry risks which should not be minimized. In my experience, the identification of the person's particular metabolic type, and any unique idiosyncracies and dysfunctions, is the first step towards health and the achievement of an ideal weight. This ideal weight may well be above what you have previously been led to believe is the desirable target. Much depends upon what nature intended for you.

One method of assessing where you ought to be in terms of weight for height is to use a chart which links these two factors together (see opposite).

When we have identified your metabolic type, and then assessed particular variations which might apply to you as a result of imbalances in one of your hormone-producing glands, we will be able to formulate a programme which will be tailored specifically to you. We will then go on to identify specific additional nutritional needs which your body has, by means of a series of questions. If answered accurately these will give a personal outline of these requirements. Before that, there are a number of important basic changes to make. These apply to everyone, and are of the utmost importance.

Most people who have repeatedly tried to lose weight will have noted one unfortunate fact. This is that, after following the particular method for a while, they begin to regain any weight loss they achieved, and frequently find themselves creeping even higher. This seems to be adding insult to injury, for it is as though the perverse nature of their weight-controlling system is over compensating for the previous attempt to lose weight. This is almost precisely what is actually happening.

After a while, at any given weight, the body adjusts itself to maintain that weight, and the complex infrastructure of circulation and nutritional supply is geared around the particular weight that is the current norm. If an attempt is made to lose swiftly some of the unwanted weight, there is a reaction by the body, which does not recognize the need for such action, and so sets about rebuilding what has been lost. Under such conditions, the efficiency of absorption and utilization of nutrients can be dramatically improved. This means that even if the diet is providing significantly less food than normal, the body can make such good use of it that it can actually gain weight.

For this reason, and those of biochemical and metabolic individuality which have been mentioned, it is my certain conviction that a slimming programme based on calorie counting is doomed from the outset. So is any programme that does anything other than provide the body with its particular and unique needs. First health, then weight adjustment. We must aim to get your body functioning well on its own ideal diet; then we will see the weight situation take care of itself.

We must provide the essential nutrients, and removed the potentially harmful non-foods, which so many people use exces-

Calculate your Body Mass

Connect a straight line from your weight to your height. Where it crosses the middle line is equal to your body mass index.

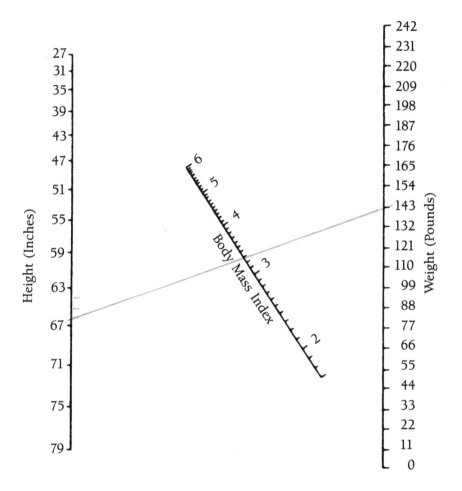

By ruling a line from your height to your weight you will cut across a point on a measure which will give you the ratio between the two figures.

This number should be between 3.2-3.7 in women, or 3.4-3.9 in men, on average. You can be perfectly normal at the top or bottom of that ratio, depending upon your metabolic type.

sively. By doing this, and reorganizing the exercise level to meet the particular needs of the body aerobically, and introducing the element of mind-participation into the programme, we have all the elements which are required for health and weight control.

Allies or enemies?

The first step is our attack on 'tasty toxins'; eliminating some undesirable components of your diet. Wherever possible, alternatives will be suggested. It is important that you do not feel deprived at the outset, and so I will explain the reasons for removing some of your favourite crutches. Once you understand the reasons for the changes they should be more easily achieved. The motivation that you have to achieve positive health and optimum weight must come into play at this stage. Once feelings of well-being and positive health begin to manifest themselves, your motivation begins to have support. In the initial stages, however, it appears that you have set out on a lonely journey without the support of your usual allies, such as coffee. Let me reassure you these are not allies, but enemies, which you are well rid of.

Put up with the minor discomforts of making alterations to the comfortable habits into which you have slipped. It is these that are holding you back from health and happiness.

How well do you eat?

Questionnaire

The following questions should be answered honestly in order to help you to identify dietary habits which may be negatively influencing your health.

Answer Yes if you are doing what the question asks more than once a week. Answer Sometimes if you are doing what the questions asks no more than once a week. Answer No if you are doing what the question asks less than once a week.

Ideally answers for questions 1-12 should be No. If there are some Yes and more than three Sometimes answers, then try to modify your habits so that next time you test the answers will be as desired, all No.

Ideally all answers for questions 13-24 should be Yes or at the very least Sometimes. Try to modify any No answers in this group to become Yes or at the very least Sometimes, the next time you assess yourself.

1. Do you eat foods made from white (refined) flour products?
2. Do you add sugar (any colour) to food or drinks?
3. Do you drink tea, coffee or cola drinks more than once daily.?
4. Is your alcohol consumption more than the equivalent of 1½ glasses wine or 1 pint of beer daily?

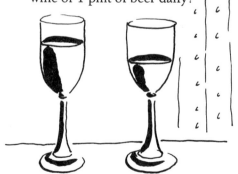

5. Do you eat food containing colouring, additives or preservatives?
6. Do you skip meals?
7. Do you eat snacks between meals?
8. Is your intake of animal protein in excess of 6 ounces daily (175 grams)?
9. Do you eat convenience foods such as TV dinners, instant mash potatoes, canned vegetables etc?

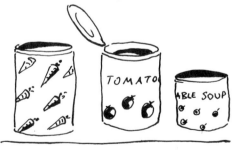

10. Do you add salt to your food at the table?
11. Do you eat fried (or very fatty) foods?
12. Do you eat smoked, preserved or pickled fish or meat?

Y 13. Do you eat fresh fruit?
N S 14. Do you eat raw vegetables (salads etc)?
Y 15. Do you insist on fresh vegetables, avoiding canned or frozen ones?
N 16. Do you use herbs for seasoning your food?
N 17. Do you make a point of ensuring a high fibre intake in your diet?
Y 18. Do you eat wholegrains such as brown rice, wholemeal bread?
N 19. Do you consume herbal teas?
N 20. Do you regularly supplement with multimineral and/or multivitamin nutrients?
N 21. Do you eat vegetable proteins such as nuts, seeds (sunflower, sesame, pumpkin etc.) or pulses (lentils, beans etc)?
Y 22. Do you eat breakfast?
N 23. Do you eat natural (live) yogurt?
N 24. Do you consume bottled or filtered rather than tap water?

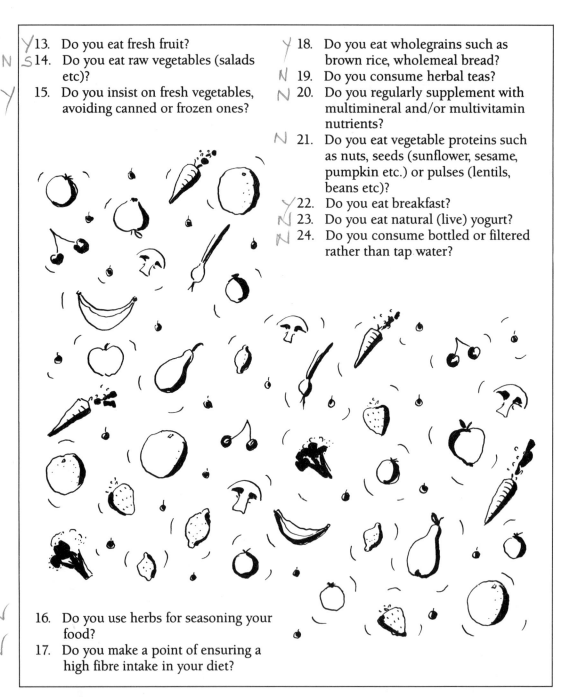

By trying to modify regular habits which conflict with the ideal as indicated by Yes answers to the first 12, and No answers to the second 12 questions, a simple method exists for enhancing general health.

Tasty toxins

Let's look at the foods and additives that we use in our daily lives which are either disturbing our normal physiological processes or which are harmful in a variety of ways. All suggestions about items which should be dropped from your diet are made for very real reasons, backed up by research evidence of potential harm and supported by my own many years of clinical experience with thousands of patients.

Remember always that you live in a body of the most amazing complexity and that it is a self-healing, self-repairing organism. You have only to provide your body with the correct inputs (balanced diet, nutrients, exercise, relaxation, etc.) and stop the negative inputs for it to function at its optimum level. Give it what it needs, stop harming it, and watch the results. If the idea of taking on this dynamic responsibility appeals to you, and you are prepared to make the first difficult sacrifices willingly, not grudgingly, then it is time to move on and consider the 'tasty toxins' of life, which have wrought such havoc to the health of the world.

Salt

Let us start with salt, which is at last receiving its just desserts at the hands of the medical fraternity. Salt (or rather, sodium) is essential to life, but we do not need to add it to our food, which already contains an adequate quantity as part of its chemical make-up. The current attention which salt is receivig world-wide as a health hazard derives from its potentially lethal effect on our blood-pressure and cardiovascular system. It has been shown that high salt intake (together with other factors, including genetic ones) is a major cause of this area of disease and consequent death. From the viewpoint of weight adjustment it is the effect of salt on the fluid balance within the body that is important. By disturbing the balance within the body of sodium and potassium, the use of salt in the diet allows a 'leaching' of fluid from the cells into what are called extra-cellular areas—fluid retention.

There are a variety of possible consequences. The most obvious result of fluid retention is, of course, a great deal of extra weight. A further, perhaps more subtle, effect of a high-salt diet is its ability to make you eat more than you actually intended, or needed. The appetite-stimulating characteristic of salt and spices, and their tendency to make you want to

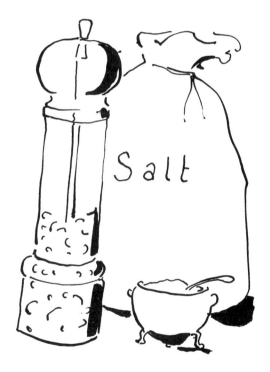

drink copious amounts of fluid, are important factors in weight reduction, over and above the health aspects.

It is possible to learn to cook with a salt substitute (potassium chloride instead of sodium chloride) which you can buy from any health store or chemist's shop, use this sparingly. The use of culinary herbs can also assist in the cutting down in the use of salt. Such herbs as oregano, sage and rosemary, as well as garlic and onion, can transform a meal far more effectively than the application of salt. If you add salt after cooking either switch to potassium chloride or, if this is not possible, block all but one of the holes in the salt shaker. This little trick has worked wonders for many salt addicts who, it has been shown, are more often addicted to the habit of sprinkling salt than to the amount of salt that emerges.

The important realization that I want you to come to is that, with this first injunction against salt, you have reached a point where you are testing your resolve about this whole enterprise. Is your desire to lose weight equalled by your commitment to that end? Are you really prepared to do something about your health and well-being? I understand all too well the feeling of not wishing to give up comfortable habits and pleasures. However the rewards are far in excess of the minor hardships inherent in the early stages of changing long held habits. So, with salt, you have your first test, and it is all up to you.

Dramatically reduce your intake, substitute herbs if you wish, and fling yourself into an adventure in self-discipline which will enrich your life and probably lengthen it, as well as adding a quality you never dreamed of.

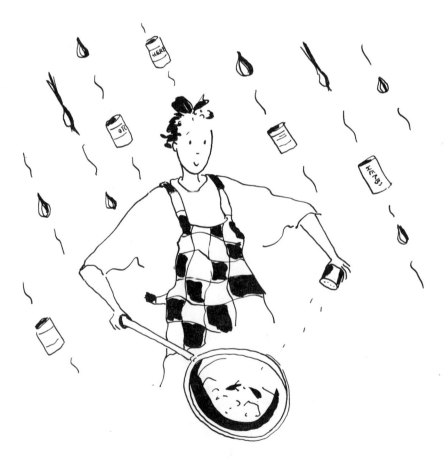

Hidden salt

Salt (sodium) is found 'hidden' in many foods (in some it is natural, in others it is added) processed meats; salami; bacon; ham; sausages; corned beef; hamburgers; smoked fish; anchovies; tinned seafood; cod roe; all cheeses, especially hard cheese and cottage cheese; milk which has been dried, evaporated or condensed; most margarines; butter; salted nuts, crisps and savoury snacks; bread, pizza, savoury biscuits, and some sweet biscuits; cornflakes, *All-bran*, and most processed breakfast foods; tinned vegetables, olives, and all vegetables preserved in brine; most stock cubes and yeast extracts; all sauces such as miso, soy, Worcester and tomato; and all foods containing baking soda.

Worst of all is added salt, such as in cooking and at table. This and cured meats and fish, and processed meats such as sausages, as well as all canned soups, meats; and vegetables and cheese, as well as additives which carry the prefix 'sodium' are to be avoided wherever possible.

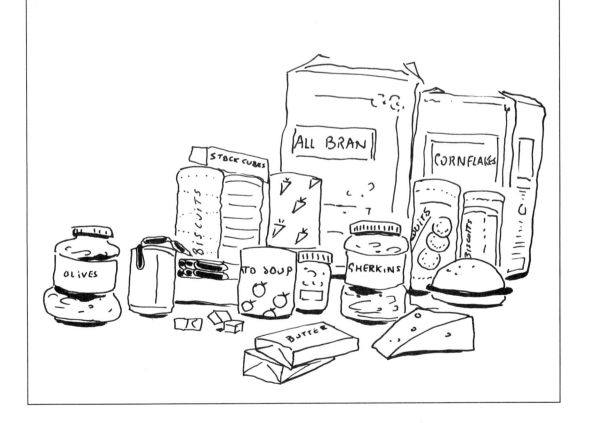

Sugar

Our next target is also white and deadly or perhaps I should qualify that statement, for it could be brown and deadly just as easily. There is no real difference nutritionally (apart from extremely low levels of trace elements) between white and brown sugar.

You actually *need* no sugar at all, and it is certainly desirable, both for health and weight control, to eliminate it from the diet. Among the health conditions now firmly connected with the use of sugar are tooth decay, diabetes, hypoglycaemia (low blood sugar), coronary disease, cancer and of course obesity. The havoc that the use of sugar plays with the appetite mechanism is so profound as to make it our greatest nutritional enemy. 'Pure, white and deadly', it has been called, and 'the curse of civilization'. Both are apt, and yet neither is sufficiently descriptive a phrase for the substance that tastes so good and yet does so much harm.

People have always been seduced by the natural sweetness of fruits, and in the very limited quantities in which sucrose (our main concern) exists in fruits, this is acceptable. The problem has arisen because the process of sugar refining has given us instant sweetness and, with it, a catalogue of physiological confusion.

When a piece of fruit is eaten the natural sugars within it (fructose, glucose, sucrose, etc.) are intimately associated with vitamins and minerals and other nutrient factors. The absorption of sugars into the blood stream is accompanied by the disappearance of hunger and a feeling of well-being. In order to metabolize sugar, all the essential nutrients necessary for processing (vitamins, minerals, some protein and fat, etc.) are required. When derived from complex carbohydrates (such as whole grains) or from fruit, some or all of these nutrients are present within the sugar.

When eaten as pure refined sugar, on its own or with other refined carbohydrates (pastry, biscuit etc.), the body has to provide these nutrients from its own stores. If refined sugar plays a large part in the diet this can lead to imbalances within the nutritional status of the individual, leading to sub-clinical deficiencies of essential food factors. The rapid appetite-placating effect of sugar has a further unfortunate result. Because sucrose is absorbed so quickly and gives so dramatic a lift to the individual, its use is associated with pleasant feelings. The truth is that this is bought at a great cost.

With the rapid rise in blood-sugar there also comes a release of a number of hormones into the system. One of these is insulin which regulates the level of blood-sugar. Because (assuming we are in a reasonable state of health), the insulin drives down the sugar level in the blood, a 'low' feeling soon replaces the previous 'high'. At this stage the individual who has become hooked into the vicious cycle will again crave (and probably have) something sweet to eat or drink, or will utilize one of the common stimulants (such as coffee, tea or cola) which encourage the production of adrenalin.

Adrenalin (also called epinephrine) brings with it a sense of strength and readiness for activity when we are stressed or excited. It also causes the release into the blood-stream of stored sugar. But many of these stimulants are, of course, laced with more copious amounts of sugar, so the process then repeats itself. Quick energy, a feeling of well-being as the blood sugar rises, followed by tiredness and edginess and a further craving for something sweet, and so on. And all the while there is an added burden of calories being absorbed which are superfluous to our needs. Weight is increasing unless the metabolism is able to cope with the onslaught, which many are not.

Digesting sugar

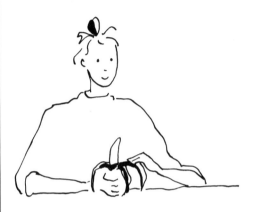

Natural sugar, i.e., fruit, provides vitamins and minerals.

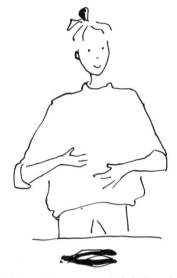

After eating, you are left feeling full and well

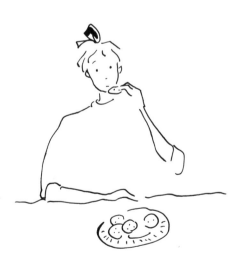

Refined sugar, i.e., cakes, provides no vitamins or minerals.

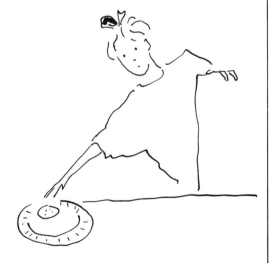

This causes a rapid rise in blood-sugar levels, followed by the release of insulin. The individual will then crave more sugary foods.

The truth is that sugar, as such, is of no value to man. We can derive all the sugar we need for our energy requirements from more complex carbohydrates such as whole cereals, fruits and vegetables. The debt we are obliged to pay for the use of sugar is far too high; physiological chaos such as nutrient deficiencies, overweight, dental decay and a catalogue of health disorders which can lead to anything from blindness (part of the diabetic legacy for many) to death.

Determine *now* that sugar will no longer seduce and corrupt you. It is the hardest step of all, for nothing else that I will ask you to do will be as vital, or as difficult, and yet so satisfying and rewarding.

It does not mean that you can never again eat anything sweet. Natural sweetness, as contained in fruits and some vegetables (carrots etc.), and the occasional use of pure honey, will be part of your programme. Refined sugar in all its myriad disguises must go, however, if we are to make the desired progress towards vital health and optimum weight reduction.

Once you have passed this stage, I promise you that you will not even consider the idea of reverting to the use of refined sugars or any of the other 'tasty toxins' we are discussing in this chapter.

I touched on the need for control of substances which replicate, to some extent, the confusion of refined sugar intake on the body, such as coffee. Other caffeine-containing substances include tea, chocolate, cola drinks, cocoa, glucose drinks, etc. There is a wide variety of herb teas and coffee substitutes which can replace these. There is also a chocolate substitute called carob. (However, there is not much point in replacing chocolate with carob if it has added sugar.)

Artificial sweeteners such as saccharine should be looked at with the gravest of suspicion since, without exception, they have come under attack from one source or another as being possible health hazards. Modest use of these is not perhaps going to have much effect on our programme, but this should not be taken as a recommendation for their use, rather as a reluctant half-concession to a need for some sweetness in the diet, other than the natural ones mentioned previously.

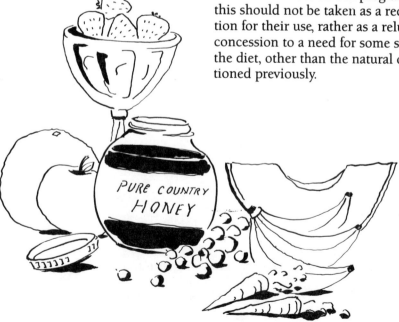

Refined foods

Remember, that the objects of this discussion of undesirable factors are twofold. First: I want them out of your diet before we try to assess your biological and metabolic individuality. Second: I want to remove from your diet factors which are going to mitigate against your long-term goal of positive health and an optimum weight level. We have so far asked that salt, sugars and stimulant-containing foods and drinks be abandoned. These are most important and the rewards you will reap from dropping these from your diet will be enormous.

Refined flour (used in white bread, cakes, pasta, biscuits, pastry, etc.) has a number of drawbacks. The refining process itself removes from the grain a variety of nutrient factors which should be associated in the body with the carbohydrate that remains. The consumption of foods which have been refined in this way creates a number of problems, not least of which is that more calories must be ingested before the appetite is satisfied.

Compare eating a slice of wholemeal bread and a slice of refined white bread, one after the other, to see that the wholemeal bread requires more chewing and takes longer to eat. This is in line with the digestive needs of the body, which require that starch digestion begins in the mouth with an adequate mixing of the food with enzymes found in saliva. The inbuilt signals with which the eating of wholefoods provide the body are in stark contrast to the confused messages which the brain receives when 'empty' calorie (refined) foods are eaten.

The calorie-rich, yet essential, unprocessed carbohydrate foods such as brown rice or wholegrain cereal products, are associated and combined in nature with substances such as fats, vitamins, minerals and enzymes which, when well chewed (as these foods demand), signal to the satiety centre in the brain that enough has been eaten, and hunger ceases. When devitalized, refined carbohydrates which have lost these associated factors are eaten, the chewing process is rapid and 'stop eating' messages to the brain are a long time coming. Thus more is eaten, and a higher calorie intake is achieved, with a consequent dual effect. The body has to yield up vital nutrients for the digestion and processing of these carbohydrates and the consequent biochemical imbalance is accompanied by increased weight.

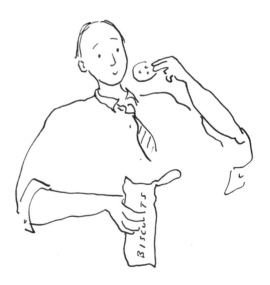

Of course, the whole range of biscuits, cakes and pastry products contain added sugar, salt and animal fats (usually) and they therefore carry double or treble negative marks, as far as our efforts are concerned.

Replace white pasta with wholemeal pasta and bread with wholewheat or rye bread, and replace white polished rice with brown unpolished rice. The taste is better and the value is undeniable.

Fats

The last food factor for us to consider is fats. It has become established that the eating of fats—any kind of fats or oils—can produce an increase in the fat deposits of the body as well as increasing the size of those fat molecules themselves. In animal experiments (and in human subjects) it was found that these effects were possible as a result of eating lard, beef fat, sunflower oil or soya oil. The eating of lard tended to increase the *number* of fat cells more than the other forms of fat, and the soya oil tended to increase the *size* of fat cells, as opposed to the other forms of fat ('Dietary-induced Obesity', *British Journal of Nutrition* 49, 17, 1983).

It was also shown that the sites at which the extra fat was laid down varied with the sex of the experimental subject. When the number of fat cells increase in a particular area the body is actually manufacturing new fat cells, as opposed to simply increasing the size of existing ones.

Typically, the fat sites that respond to new fat-cell deposits in females are those surrounding the genital organs (hips and lower abdomen) leading to the traditional 'pear shape' figure. Now it is not always easy to relate experimental evidence in animals to the human model, but the fact remains that it appears to confirm the well-known observation that the eating of fats and oils induces obesity (as well as coronary disease and cancer) and that different forms of fats and oils produce different types of fat deposits, in different sexes, at different ages.

The overall conclusion indicates that the less fat contained in your diet the better, and the less of this fat that is made up of animal fats, the less chance of forming new fat cells. It is patently easier to reduce the overall cell size by dietary measures than it

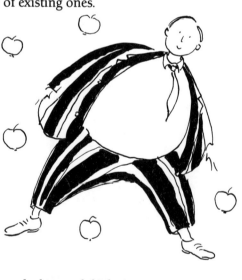

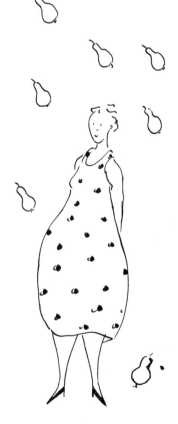

Fat deposits on the hips and thighs in women can lead to the traditional pear-shaped figure. Men may find a more even spread of fat produces an apple-shaped physique.

is to reduce the number of fat cells present in any particular area of the body.

The type of oil or fat that is available to the body in the diet is important to the general economy of the cells of the body, in particular, and to the body as a whole, in general. As our marvellous bodies evolved, nature assumed that the fats we would eat (and, for that matter, the sugars) would be associated in their consumption and digestion with all the B vitamins, vitamin C, all the essential minerals (20 or so), as well as other nutrient factors of which we as yet know little. In fact without these, *all of these*, we cannot digest one single molecule of fat or sugar.

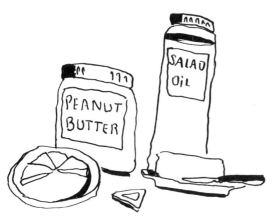

By consuming quantities of concentrated fats and oils (think of margarine, butter, peanut butter, processed cheese, salad oils, pastries containing lard and hydrogenated oils, etc.) we disrupt the designed intention of the body and create imbalances. Evidence is strong that this creates interference with cell membrane function and cholesterol transport (*American Journal of Nutrition* 30, 1009-1017). This has been described as 'a major disaster (for the cell) because fat molecules no longer come in the shape and size they (the cells) have become accustomed to over the last 10 million years.'

Weight control

There are people who eat enormous quantities of foods which should, but do not, make them fat. There are others, and perhaps you are one of them, who eat hardly at all but for whom life is a constant battle with a weight problem. This highlights what I have already stated about individuality. It also helps me to make the point that eating, or not eating, particularly undesirable foods matters greatly, whether or not there is an obvious weight problem. As mentioned above the consumption of concentrated sugars and fats produces stresses on the physiological processes which are potentially devastating, even fatal. Cancer has been estimated by experts to be 40 per cent the result of dietary factors. I would put it much higher, and the key dietary culprits are, unsurprisingly, salt, refined carbohydrates, fats and chemicalized foods. So whether ot not what you eat makes you fat it certainly determines, to a large extent, how healthy you are.

Fats, especially saturated fats, animal fats and any processed oils, are undesirable to the point where they should play no part in your eating pattern at all. Our aim is a new healthy, trim-style you. That picture in your mind should be a beacon, leading you on, and the abandoned habits littering your path are milestones of achievement. If we look at the controversies which rage in scientific circles regarding the whole question of weight gain and weight control, we can learn some interesting facts.

Firstly we learn that the thin person who apparently eats a great deal without affecting his or her weight 'burns off' the excess weight. The term 'luxisconsumption' was coined to describe the observation that a normal individual who eats more than his requirements for maintaining weight, will, after an initial weight gain, establish a new weight-level, which his body will maintain by somehow disposing of the extra energy. What happens to that extra energy, since it is not stored as fat, is a source of much research (*British Medical Journal,* vol 1286, 1983).

Fascinatingly, if you measure the resting energy output of a thin person as well as a fat one you find that the thin one is 'burning' more energy. If you feed them both on a variety of foods and then again measure their energy output at rest, some strange facts emerge. Overall the comparison shows that the energy output of the fat person is *higher* than the thin person. It is generally agreed that certain very specific areas of fatty deposit are what is termed 'brown' fat cells. These areas are where heat production or thermogenesis (the burning of excess energy without actual exercise) takes place. Some individuals' brown fat cells have a higher rate of activity than those of others.

Research tells us that genetic factors play a large part in the whole process (which we already knew of course) but also that aerobic exercise and a nutritionally correct wholefood diet can help promote the functioning of under-active brown fat cells.

There is another piece of scientific research which is of relevance to us in our quest for the optimum weight control plan. It was found possible to 'programme' laboratory animals to overeat by exposing them to what is termed 'tasty cafeteria' type food, instead of their normal monotonous laboratory 'chow', which was nutritionally correct but rather uninteresting.

What we can learn from this is that to some extent we must reduce the artificially stimulating quality of our food, if we are to avoid overeating. This does not mean that food need be dull, but that the use of highly processed, flavoured, commercially-prepared foods are best avoided if we are to avoid falling into the trap of over-indulgence to satisfy the jaded palate. The last change to our dietary pattern at this stage of the programme is, therefore, the avoidance of the use of foods which have been artificially chemicalized to enhance flavour. This rules out prepacked convenience foods (also high in salt, sugar and saturated fats).

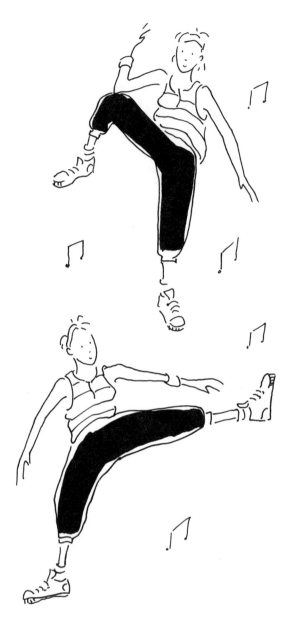

Items to avoid

Let us summarize what we are giving up, or rather what we are releasing ourselves from, in order to begin the process of health achievement and weight adjustment.

Salt
No more than ½ teaspoon daily (5 grams). This means avoiding anything to which salt is added. Replace with potassium chloride.

Sugar
None at all, if possible. Two teaspoons of unprocessed honey daily, for sweetening, if absolutely necessary.

Tea, coffee, chocolate
Replace with herb tea, carob (sugarless) and coffee substitutes.

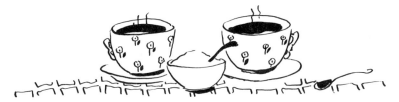

Fats
Reduce use of oil to include limited quantity of virgin olive oil (2 tablespoons daily) or pure sunflower oil (2 tablespoons daily). Avoid processed cheese, full-fat milk, full-fat cheese, butter and margarine, muscle meats (contain up to 30 per cent fat), lard, shortening. Use low-fat cheese and skimmed milk and no more than ½ oz (15g/1 tablespoon) unsalted butter daily.

White flour products
Replace with wholemeal flour products (pasta, bread, etc.).

White rice
Use unpolished rice or millet instead.

Convenience flavoured factory food
Avoid completely.

Cured, salted, pickled or preserved meat or fish
Avoid completely.

These first essential steps will, in themselves make a dramatic change in your metabolism and well-being.

You should expect changes in your bowel function (more frequent) and perhaps be prepared for some mild skin eruptions in the first weeks of change. The body eliminates impurities and toxic accumulations via any convenient channel, so there is sometimes an outbreak, or redness, on the skin or a mild looseness of the bowel for a few days. All this will rapidly normalize and should be seen as a sign of the adjustment of the body to its new regime.

You should also start to sleep better and, once you have overcome the withdrawal from stimulants, you will find that you feel far more energetic and less nervous.

Don't start on this programme, however, until you have begun a basic nutrition supplementation programme of 3 brewer's yeast tablets with each meal (a total of 9 daily). This gives you the essential B vitamins and certain minerals (e.g., selenium and chromium) which are important in the economy of the body and which will help during the transition stage until we have identified your particular nutritional needs.

Continue with this pattern until you indentify your metabolic type, when more specific nutrients may be seen to apply to your need. The general interim pattern of diet for the period, during which you are assessing your particular nutritional needs should be within the framework of the following guidelines.

This is an arbitrary pattern which excludes the substances as discussed above, and yet which does not take into account individual metabolic idiosyncracies, which we have yet to assess.

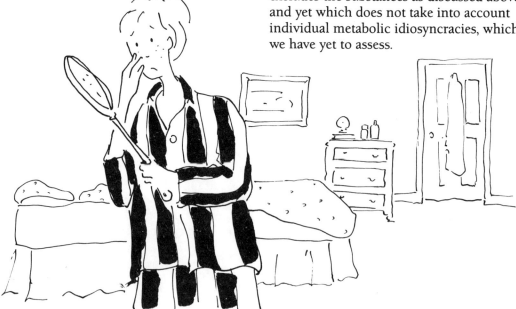

The experienced slimmer will by now have realized that the word fibre has hardly appeared in this book. The reason for this is that the pattern we will work towards contains fibre as naturally as eggs contain protein. It is not something you will have to concern yourself with for, by removing the 'tasty toxins', and reducing your salt and fat intake to acceptable limits, the foods that are left (and they are many and varied) will provide all the fibre you need.

The basic dietary pattern
Breakfast pattern

Choose from the following (or, if appetite dictates, eat all of them):

● One or two slices of wholemeal or rye bread or toast. A scraping of unsalted butter plus 2-3 oz (55-85g ¼-⅓ cup) cottage cheese (add any green salad you fancy such as cress or lettuce—optional).

● Dried fruit which has been soaked in water overnight or lightly cooked (no sweetening) plus low-fat natural yogurt. Add all or any of the following: 2 teaspoons wheatgerm; 2 teaspoons linseed (from health store); sprinkling of sunflower or pumpkin seeds.

● 2 oz (55g/½ cup) oatmeal porridge, made with water or skimmed milk. Add powdered (in a food processor) almonds (1 oz/25 g/¼ cup) or sprinkle sunflower or pumpkin seeds.

● One or two items fresh fruit (skin as well if edible).

● Home made muesli plus low-fat natural yogurt or unsweetened fruit juice.

● Herb tea or china tea or coffee substitute.

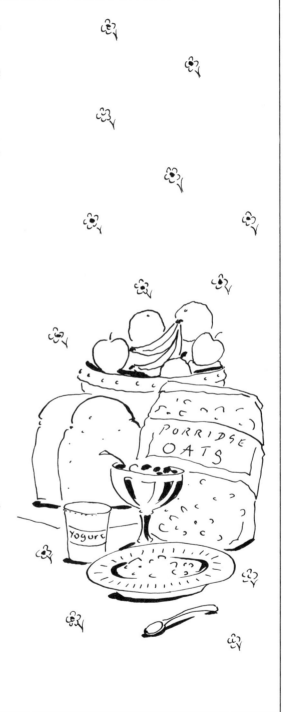

Lunch

One of the main meals each day should be constructed around a mixed raw salad.

We will assume that it is the midday meal for the purpose of this menu:

Mixed salad to include whatever is seasonally available. Shred and mix and dress (a little olive oil, natural yogurt, lemon juice and a touch of honey make a fantastic dressing) and serve with either baked jacket potato or boiled brown rice or boiled millet (see recipe section). Only 1 oz (25g/¼ cup) of either low-fat cheese or fish is allowable.

The salad should be varied and should contain at least two green vegetables (water-cress, pepper, mustard and cress, lettuce, chicory, endive, cabbage, celery, etc.) as well as a root vegetable finely shredded (raw beetroot/beet, carrot, etc.) and tomato, sliced mushroom, radish, etc.

In total never try to have less than four salad ingredients, of which at least one is a root vegetable. Obviously, more variety is acceptable but the main thing is to make it interesting by varying the colours, textures and tastes of the ingredients. Low-fat cheese can include cottage, Feta or Edam.

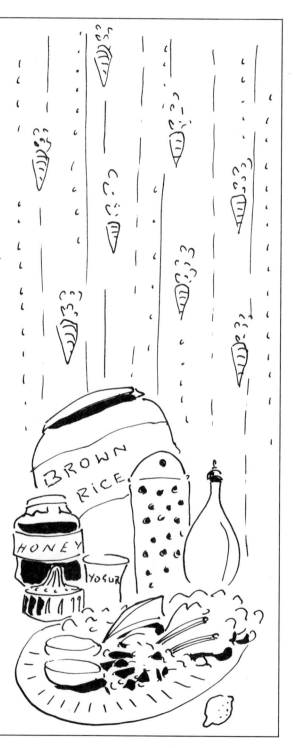

Evening meal

This should comprise:
4 ounces (115g) of protein such as fish, egg, lean meat or organ meat (liver etc.) or chicken (no skin) or a vegetarian bean-and-cereal mixture plus a variety of raw or cooked vegetables. None of this should be fried in oil or fat. Stir-frying in a wok, or its equivalent, is acceptable however.

Desserts should be of fresh fruit, or low-fat yogurt or dried fruit or sunflower or pumpkin seeds.

Up to 1½ wineglasses of wine may be taken with one of your meals without endangering the programme.

The diet, as outlined, gives enormous scope and variety and you should never find any difficulty in ringing the changes and yet remain within the guidelines.

Never eat between meals. If you are desperate for a snack have some natural yogurt or unsweetened fruit juice or *Perrier* water.

Once we have established what your particular biological and metabolic needs are, the pattern outlined above will probably require modification to suit those needs. For the time being however you will find the pattern nutritious and satisfying. Do not forget to take three brewer's yeast tablets with each meal.

After a few transition days, during which you may have withdrawal symptoms from your previous habits (coffee, etc.), you should find all, or some, of the following benefits from this pattern of eating:
- you should be more relaxed and energetic
- sleeping better
- with digestion and bowels better than in years
- some slight weight reduction (probably not more than 3 pounds/1.5 kilos a week in the first few weeks).

Your main benefits will not be manifesting themselves yet as you have not started providing the nutrients your biological individuality demands.

Eating

In addition to making the suggested changes in your pattern of eating there are also a number of simple, yet important, aspects relating to the very act of eating which require attention.

Since digestion actually begins in the mouth, and since this is part of a complex process which keeps your brain informed as to what and how much you are eating, it is important actually to chew your food. This may seem self-evident, but it is amazing to discover just how lax people are over this. If you chew well (until the food in your mouth is reduced to a creamy texture) before swallowing, then it will be well mixed with the enzymes present in your saliva, and digestion will be more efficient.

If you eat very 'mushy' or 'pappy' foods which require little chewing, you are likely to swallow the food long before such essential mixing has taken place. It is therefore advisable to eat most of your food in a state which requires a lot of chewing. Crisp, crunchy chewable foods, such as salads, fruits, wholegrain products, nuts and seeds, all fall into this category.

Sauces and relishes, besides containing undesirable substances, such as salt, sugar and sometimes artificial flavourings, have the effect of stimulating appetite, which is one more good reason for avoiding them.

It has long been known that, if a person is upset or angry, their digestive function is seriously impaired. If you should feel distressed or angry at a meal time you would do far better to skip the meal and have a walk or a rest rather than eat for the sake of eating. Try to practise the relaxation methods that you will learn in the later chapters, or go for a pleasant walk, and eat later when you are calmer. You will be doing yourself, and your digestive system a favour. Missing a meal or two never did any harm at all.

Fitness and relaxation

Questionnaire

The answers to the following questions will give you some general guidance as to your level of stress and the degree of exercise.

As in the dietary questionnare in the last chapter the answers to the following questions will increase your awareness of what is needed in terms of change.

The questions should all be answered Yes. Any No answers indicate a need for change.

1. Do you ensure that your main meals are leisurely, taking at least half an hour?

2. Do you ensure that you do not work for more than 10 hours on work days?

3. Do you ensure that you do not work more than 5½ days weekly?

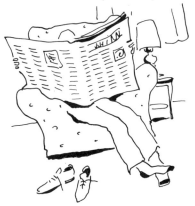

4. Do you ensure that you have not less than 2 weeks complete holiday from work annually?

5. Do you avoid eating rapidly or chewing inadequately?

6. Do you avoid smoking?

7. Do you ensure that you sleep not less than 7 hours nightly?

8. Do you regularly walk rather than drive on journeys under a mile?

9. Do you try to avoid having more than one major task on hand at a time?

10. Do you try to avoid deadlines and pressure in your work by allowing adequate time and working methodically?

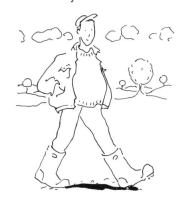

11. Do you practise relaxation or meditation?

12. Do you take not less than 30 minutes active exercise three times weekly?

13. Do you have a hobby which is creative (gardening, painting, etc.)?

14. Do you participate in non-competitive sports such as walking, cycling, swimming, or belong to a yoga or exercise class?

15. Do you ensure a short siesta during the day?

16. Do you listen to relaxing music?

17. Do you have regular massage, bodywork or osteopathic treatment?

18. Do you spend at least half an hour outdoors daily in fresh air and daylight?

19. Do you take an interest in other people, world and local events and in improving environmental conditions?

20. Do you try to hug someone at least once a day?

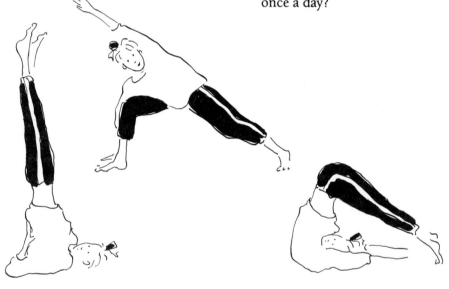

The answers to these questions should be Yes in every instance and any that produce No as an answer might give you pause to think about the quality of your life and the degree of frenzy attached to it.

Regular exercise, pleasant work habits, adequate rest, involvement with society's needs and with those of other people, all add to the quality of living and make a contribution at least as important as dietary factors.

Exercise

Before considering the subject of biological individuality it is necessary to give some general guidance on the exercise and relaxation methods which should accompany you on the journey towards positive health and weight adjustment.

Exercise is necessary to maintain and to improve general function. A variety of different methods is the ideal. Some should be designed to:
- stretch our bodies,
- some should tone up and increase our circulatory and respiratory efficiency,
- and some should be to relax us.

Wherever possible, any given exercise session should carry with it components of all these aspects of exercise—stretch, tone, relax.

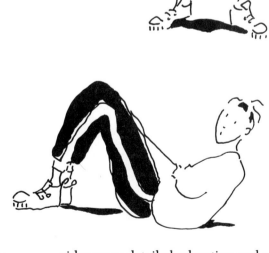

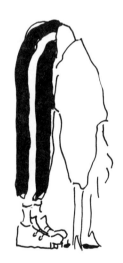

At this stage it is not necessary to do more than to begin a habitual daily 20 minute session during which the simplest of these methods will be introduced. Consider more detailed relaxation and exercise (chapter 6) once you have used the introductory pattern for a month or so.

Introductory stretching exercises

These exercises are meant to produce general effects. To start with do the following movements three times each. After a few days increase them to ten times each.

Exercise 1

Stand up straight with your feet apart and your hands clasped behind your back.

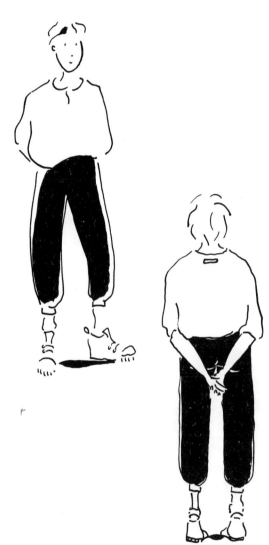

Allow yourself to bend forward from the hips as far as is comfortable. Use no effort but try to allow the weight of the upper body to stretch you forwards. Feel the stretch up the back of your legs and especially behind the knees. This exercise is not repeated. You simply hold the position for half a minute, at first breathing slowly and deeply, and allowing the stretch to reach its maximum.

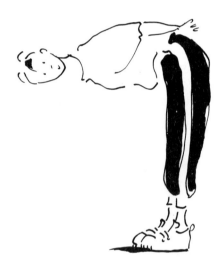

As the days go by allow the time in this position to increase to three minutes. This stretches the hamstrings; helps the muscular supporting structures of the pelvis, and improves abdominal tone if you breath slowly and deeply all the while.

Exercise 2

You may, at first, need to hold onto a solid object such as a heavy table to do this movement without losing balance. If you can do it unaided, so much the better.

With your feet about 12 to 15 inches (30 to 38cm) apart and standing up straight slowly go into a squatting position, trying to keep your heels on the floor.

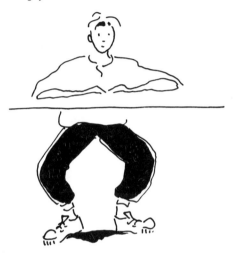

If this is not possible then either go just as far as you can into the squat without raising your heels, or wear high heels when doing this exercise.

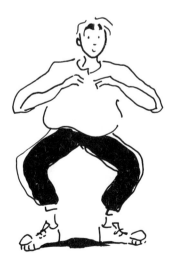

As you squat, stretch your arms forward and lean forward from the waist to maintain balance. If you feel you are toppling backwards you may need to use your hands to balance by holding onto a table or some other heavy object.

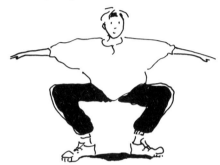

When you are at the fullest limit of your squat give a few gentle up and down 'jigs' as though you are trying to tuck your tail between your legs. Rise and repeat.

The object of this is to tone the hamstrings but also to act as a general stimulant to circulation and muscle tone in the pelvic area, and to stretch the lower back.

When this becomes easy to perform you can vary it by using the more advanced technique of interlocking the fingers behind the neck as you start (head facing straight ahead.) At the end of each deep squat rise to your feet slowly, and as you do stretch the hands (still interlocked) towards the ceiling pressing open palms as far upwards as possible. This is further enhanced by breathing in deeply as you stretch upwards. Repeat three to ten times.

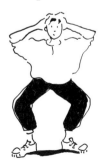

Exercise 3

The following variations on chair exercises are designed to achieve general stretching of the upper body, without strain.

First, sit on an ordinary dining chair, feet together and hands clasped behind the back. Bend forward from the waist with the hands stretching backwards and upwards as far as you can. Your trunk should be leaning forward, as far as you can, so that your nose is as close to your knees as it can get. The hands should stretch up and back and be held there for five to ten seconds as you breathe in and out. Sit up and repeat.

After doing this a number of times separate your feet so that there is a wide gap between your knees. Repeat the exercise but, instead of bending straight forwards, bend instead towards each knee alternately.

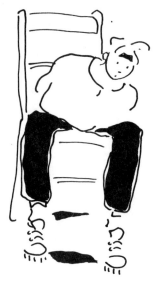

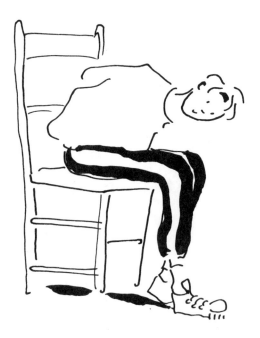

This time keep the hands clasped behind the back without stretching them backwards. Repeat several times in each direction, holding for a full cycle of breathing.

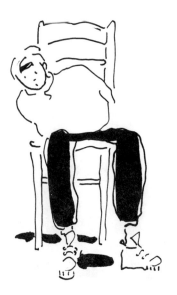

Exercise 4

Sit straight up in the chair, feet together and arms extended sideways, palms downwards. Breathe in and turn the palms upwards and at the same time stretch the arms backwards so that you feel the shoulder blades coming towards each other. Relax and breathe out as the arms resume their original position. Repeat.

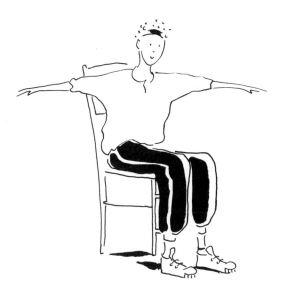

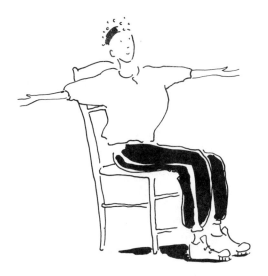

Exercise 5

Sitting, place your hands behind your neck, or rest the fingertips on the shoulders, whichever is more comfortable. Slowly rotate the shoulders so that the arms are moving in a large gentle circle (as though you are drawing circles with your elbows).

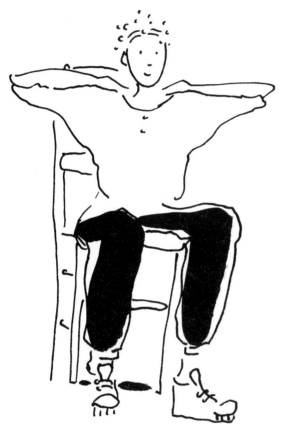

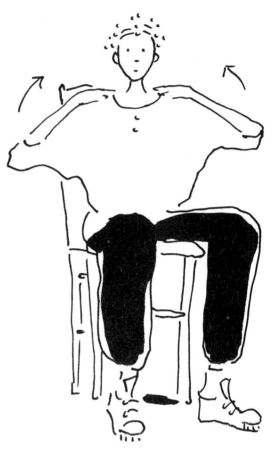

Repeat in each direction several times. You should try to achieve maximum stretch as the elbows circle, so that they go back, then down, then forward, then up as far as possible in each direction of circling.

These five exercises are the basic introduction to stretching and mobilizing the tight parts of the body. Do them once daily at least; twice daily if possible. Do not do them after a meal, allow at least an hour and a half after eating. Preferably do them alone, in a relaxed atmosphere.

As well as this, at this stage, your only other commitment to exercise is to walk each day, as briskly as you can, for at least five and preferably ten minutes. It is not necessary to take pulse rates at this stage. Simply get used to regular movement within your normal limits. Don't jog, just walk briskly, trying to keep a regular pattern of deep breathing going if you can.

Relaxation

Whilst learning the technique, arrange to have two free periods per day, each of five to fifteen minutes. Find a quiet room where you know you will not be disturbed. Rest on your back, head and shoulders slightly raised, pillows under the knees to take the strain off them and off your back. Rest your hands on the upper abdomen, close your eyes, settle down in a comfortable position.

Ensure that there is nothing in the way to distract your attention, such as sunlight, a clock, animals and so on. Sitting in a reclining position is also suitable, and many people prefer this to lying down. Try both, and choose whichever is most comfortable.

First tense and relax each part of the body in turn to ensure you are free of tension (see pages 44-45).

Correct breathing is also of great value in relaxation, particularly during the initial stages. The person who is at ease with himself and the world breathes slowly, deeply and rhythmically. Breathing is the only automatic function which one is capable of controlling. It is partly carried out through the autonomic nervous system and partly through the central nervous system. The autonomic nervous system is that which controls vital functions, endocrine (hormone) secretions and emotions. By controlling one's breathing, one can influence all these and, for a short time, take over conscious responsibility for them.

The aim is to breathe slowly, deeply and rhythmically. You cannot expect to do this perfectly to begin with—it might even take weeks. Inhale through the nose slowly and deeply. The abdomen, on which the hands are resting, should rise gently as the breathing begins. An awareness of this rising and falling of the abdomen is important to establish that the diaphragm is being used properly.

The inhalation should be slow, unforced and unhurried. Whilst breathing in, silently and slowly, count to four, five or six. When the inhalation is complete, pause for two or three seconds, then slowly exhale through the nose. As you exhale, you should feel the abdomen slowly descend. Count this breathing out, as you did when breathing in. (Again a count of four, five or six should be achieved.) *The exhalation should take at least as long as the inhalation.*

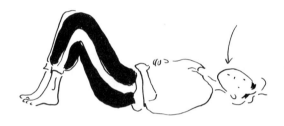

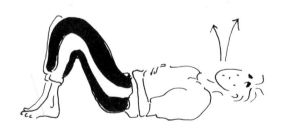

Continued on page 46

Relaxation techniques

Lift your right hand an inch off the floor. Make a fist and tense the muscles in your arm. Relax and drop it down again. Repeat with other arm.

Hunch your shoulders up around your neck. Lift them off the floor, hold and then relax. Pull in each arm alongside the body and relax.

After tensing each part of your body, let your mind command each part to relax. Just let yourself go.

Lift your right foot an inch off the floor, tense the muscles in the leg, hold and then let it drop. Repeat with other foot.

Clench your buttocks together, lift your hips off the floor and hold. Then relax and drop down again.

Keeping your hips and head on the floor, tighten your chest and lift up your back. Relax and drop down again.

Tighten every muscle in your face, as if you are trying to touch your nose with your face.

Tuck in your chin and roll your head from side to side. Find a comfortable, central position and then relax.

Now stretch your face open, with your eyes open and stick your tongue out as far as it will go. Relax.

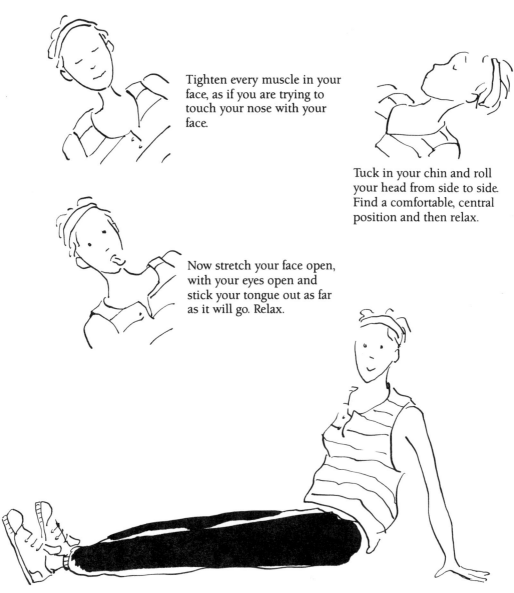

When you want to return to consciousness, gently move your fingers and toes, take a deep breath and sit up as you exhale.

Continued from page 43

There should be no sense of strain regarding the breathing cycle. If, at first, you feel you have breathed to your fullest capacity by a count of three, then so be it. Gradually try to slow down the rhythm until a slow count of five or six is possible, both on inhalation and exhalation, with a pause of two or three seconds between each change. Remember to start each breath with an upward push of the abdomen.

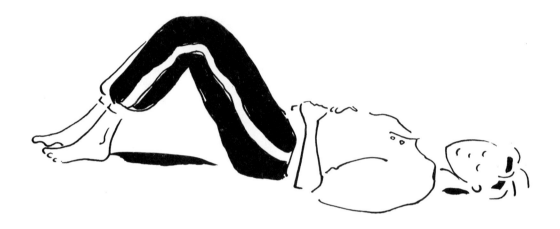

With the mind thus occupied on the mechanics of breathing and the rhythmic counting, there is little scope for thinking about anything else. Nevertheless, initially at least, extraneous thoughts will intrude. This pattern of breathing should be repeated 15 to 20 times and, since each cycle should take about 15 seconds, this exercise should occupy a total of about five minutes.

During the exercise, once the mechanics and counting have become well established as a pattern, it is useful to introduce a pattern of thoughts during different phases of the cycle. For example, on inhalation, try to sense a feeling of warmth and energy entering the body with the air. On exhaling, sense a feeling of sinking and settling deeper into the supporting surface. An overall sense of warmth and heaviness accompanying the repetitive breathing cycle will effectively begin the relaxation process.

Physiologically, this exercise will slow down the heart rate, reduce sympathetic nervous activity, relax tense muscles and allow a chance for the balancing, restorative, parasympathetic nervous function to operate, as well as calming the mind.

In the initial stages, this might be sufficient exercise for one session.

After completion of the exercise do not get up immediately. Rest for a minute or two, allowing the mind to become aware of any sensations of stillness, warmth, heaviness, etc. Once mastered, this exercise can be used in any tense situation with the certainty that it will defuse the normal agitated response and should result in a far greater ability to cope.

What is your metabolic type?

Our first task is to try to discover, from a variety of signs and indications, some of which you may never have considered, whether or not your metabolism requires assistance in our task of health and weight adjustment.

The task of uncovering the true individual nature of your biochemical and metabolic make-up should not be undertaken if you are someone who is overly obsessed by health matters. I do not want you to be constantly looking at every aspect of health and trying to deduce from odd changes that this or that hormone gland is over or under functioning.

Just carry out the tests as directed; fill in the questionnaires dealing with health appraisal and follow the appropriate advice that stems from the results. Then forget about the tests and questions for at least six months (unless I indicate otherwise) at which time a reassessment is valid. In other words, we are trying to solve your health problems and adjust your weight to its optimum, not create a person so involved in the minutiae of their health that they forget that the prime purpose of all this is to be happy, and to get on with the job of living a full life.

Temperature reading

The first little test is simplicity itself. Before getting out of bed in the morning, and before having anything to eat or drink (even water), place a normal, body thermometer, under one of your arms (touching the skin) and leave it there for exactly ten minutes. Take the reading and write this down. Do this for three mornings in a row and take the average (that is, add the three temperatures together, and divide by three). If you are a woman, and are still menstruating, then I suggest you start this procedure on the second morning of your period.

If the result (average of three days) is below 97.8°F (36.55°C) then the indication is that you have an underactive thyroid function.

If the temperature averages above 98.2°F (36.8°C) then the indication is that you have an overactive thyroid function.

Between the two indicates normal thyroid function.

When we have completed all the other assessments, we will decide just what this means in terms of your programme. For the moment just record this fact in a notebook, which I suggest you keep to record some of the pertinent results and instructions resulting from our quest.

> *Note:* By the time you have undertaken this test and any subsequent ones you should have been following the detoxification diet (previous chapter) and the introductory exercise and relaxation programme for at least two weeks.

Adrenal blood-pressure test

If you have access to a blood-pressure test, there is a check which is designed to indicate underactive adrenal function. This, together with the thyroid test, will help us ascertain whether you have any particular hormonal dysfunctions which, together with the assessments of your 'type' characteristics, gives us much of the necessary information to make suggestions unique to your needs.

Blood-pressure is taken after lying down for four minutes, and then again immediately on standing up. If the higher of the two figures in the readings (the systolic pressure) is not five to ten points higher in the standing reading, then there is considered to be adrenal underfunction. This can be the case, whatever the dominant feature of your assessment is.

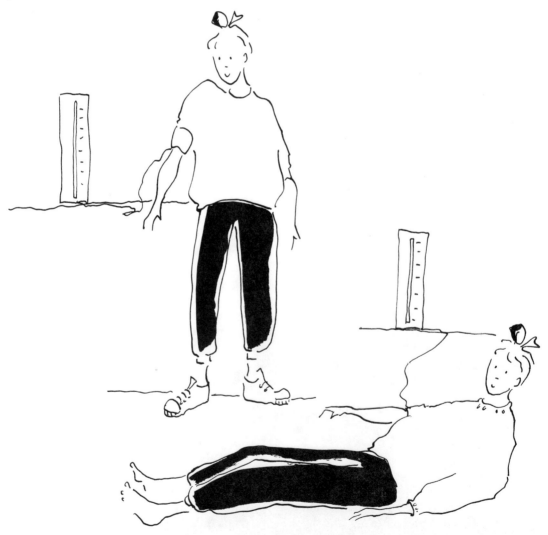

Fitness index

It is now time to calculate your fitness index. Once again, we start with you in bed before rising. As soon as you can after awaking, take your pulse for one minute and record the result. Try to do this for a number of consecutive mornings (at least three) and record the results and arrive at an average (add the numbers recorded together and then divide by the number of days that you took the pulse). The average could be anywhere between 40 and 100.

The next stage is to do some arithmetic. Write down the number 220 and deduct your age from this. Then deduct from the remainder your average morning pulse rate.

This leaves you with a subtotal which we can use to calculate two numbers which will be important to your exercise programme. You must calculate what 60 per cent ($3/5$) and 80 per cent ($4/5$) of the subtotal are. You then add back to those figures the morning pulse rate and we now have two numbers which indicate the pulse rate limits we wish to achieve in our exercise programme. These are the limits which, if you exceed the higher figure (as evidenced by your exercising pulse rate) put you in danger of stressing yourself; and if you remain below the lower figure indicates that you are not achieving much in the way of fitness.

The length of time that you keep the pulse rate above the lower figure should increase. At first, half a minute is adequate, but after a few weeks this should gradually be raised to five minutes daily whenever you are doing active aerobic exercises. At no time should the pulse rate be allowed to rise above the upper limit, set by the higher number.

You can learn to test your pulse rate during exercise without having to stop, by simply taking it for ten seconds and multiplying by six. All this will become clearer as we discuss specific exercises for your particular needs in the appropriate chapter. At this stage all we need to know is your unique limits as far as exercise is concerned, and the mathematical calculations, as set out above, will give you these guidelines.

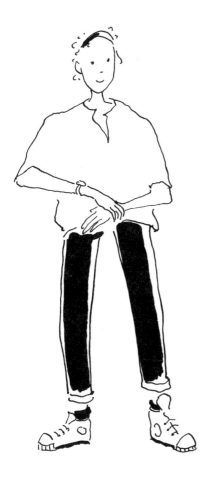

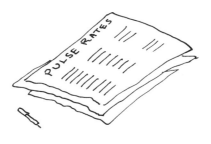

Pulse rates and fitness index

220 − your age (e.g. 40) = 180

180 − resting morning pulse (e.g. 66) = 114

60% of 114 = 68

80% of 114 = 91

Add back the resting morning pulse (e.g. 66) = 134 and 157

Try to keep your exercising pulse rate between these two figures.

Now as you get fitter, say after a few months on the diet and exercise programme, you can reassess your morning resting pulse rate and you should find that it has dropped. So if it was 66 it may now be 60. If there has been a change in rate it means that it is time to recalculate your limits, as you will have increased the range above which harm could be caused by activity. This is a marvellous way of proving to yourself that you are really getting fitter and healthier.

Do remember that the example given should not simply be copied, it requires that you use *your* age and *your* morning pulse rate in the sums. Record the two key numbers in your notebook for future reference. We have got your thyroid and adrenal indication and your fitness index numbers, and it is now time to answer a number of questions which will tell us more about yourself.

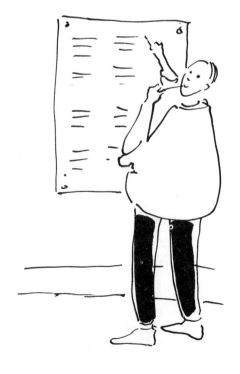

Questionnaire

What we are trying to identify, at this stage, is into which of a number of categories or 'types' you fit. Different researchers have used different criteria to help in such identification, and we will use an amalgam of their methods and ideas in order to arrive at a broad classification. It should be explained that few of us are totally one 'type'. We are more often a mix of several aspects of all the types, but usually with one more prominent than the others. The names, or labels which have been given to these types vary with the particular researcher.

What Dr William Kelley (*One Answer to Cancer*) calls his 'sympathetic-vegetarian type', comes close to what Dr Henry Bieler (*Food is Your Best Medicine*) calls his 'pituitary type'. Kelley's 'parasympathetic-carnivore type' appears to equate with Bielers 'adrenal type' and so on. There are other classifications, such as Sheldon's, in which people are typed according to physical characteristics.

For example, **endomorphs** are soft, round people with large abdomens;

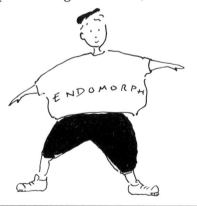

mesomorphs are square, firm people with large muscles and bones;

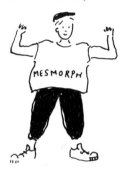

and **ectomorphs** are tall, fragile people with long extremities.

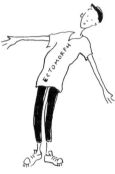

It is possible to link all these different methods (and others) of classification together, and to arrive at a way of defining your particular place in the scheme of things, and to deduce from that some of your particular nutritional and exercise requirements. By answering the series of questions, as accurately as possible, you will find what mixture of characteristics exist in you and which sort of metabolism you have.

Scoring

Answer the questions with a tick (✓), cross (x) or a question mark (?), to indicate respectively 'yes', 'no' and 'sometimes'. In terms of time, 'sometimes' means less than once a week and more than once a month. If less than once a month then score as a 'no'. 'Yes' should mean always or at least once a week.

Thyroid metabolism questionnaire

1. Are you constipated?

2. Do you have problems with your sleep?

3. Do you enjoy cool weather?

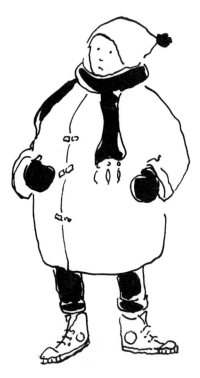

4. Do you 'catch' bacterial infections relatively easily?

5. Would you describe yourself as restless and/or very quick-thinking?

6. Are your features delicate or fine?

7. Is sex exquisitely pleasurable to you?

8. Do you wake fresh in the morning?

9. Do you sweat easily?

10. Is your hair silky or fine?

11. Do you have an easily upset digestion, preferring small snacks to large set meals?

12. Do you enjoy eating salads and vegetables?

13. Do you get tired easily, or feel a need for quiet periods by yourself?

14. Do you react quickly to stress and emotional upsets?

15. Are you very sensitive to pain?

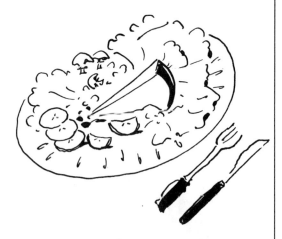

Score one point for each 'yes' and a half point for each 'sometimes' and nothing for a 'no'.

At this stage just jot down your score and we will compare it with the scores in the following assessments.

Pituitary metabolism questionnaire

1. Do you have a daily bowel movement?

2. Do you fall asleep easily at night?

3. Are your limbs long and loose jointed (perhaps with a proneness to flat feet or knock knees)?

4. Do you find it difficult to stay faithful to only one partner in affairs of the heart?

5. Would you describe your appetite as normal (rather than very small or enormous)?

6. Do you use tea, coffee or alcohol to help to 'keep you going' or to give you a lift?

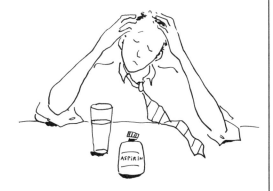

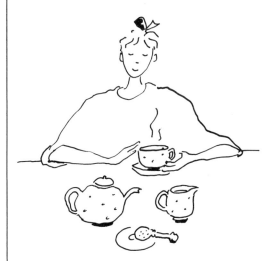

7. Are you sometimes described as idealistic, or 'a bit of a dreamer'?

8. Do you rely on intuition in making decisions?

9. Is your sexual drive strong?

10. Are you prone to headaches?

11. Do you have a good pain tolerance level?

12. Do you dislike salted food?

13. Do you have marked periods of activity interspersed with times of depression and inability to work?

14. Are you considered creative or artistic?

15. Do you have long thin supple fingers and/or well formed moons on your nails?

Scoring one point for a 'yes' and half for a 'sometimes' and none for a 'no', you will arrive at a score which you should note down for future reference.

Adrenal metabolism questionnaire

1. Do you have more than one bowel movement daily?

2. Is your digestion so good that you can eat almost anything without discomfort?

3. Are your hands and feet normally warm?

4. Have you well developed muscles?

5. When you cut yourself does your blood clot very quickly?

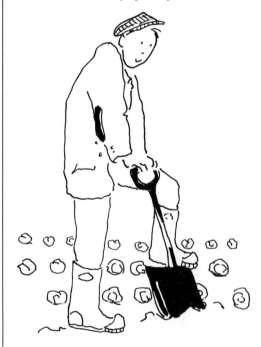

6. Have you a lot of stamina (seldom physically tired), and do you really enjoy physical work?

7. Are you slow to anger (easy to live with)?

8. Is eating one of the great pleasures of your life?

9. Do you enjoy eating meat and feel well after doing so?

10. Has your face a good colour and/or does it flush easily?

11. Are your fingers on the short side?

12. Do you crave or particularly like salty food?

13. Do you make decisions only after full deliberation and thought?

14. If naturally tired from a hard day's work are you unlikely to be easily aroused sexually?

15. Have you particularly good teeth, resistant to decay?

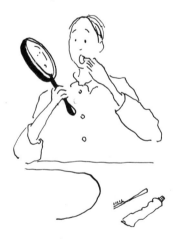

Answers, as with the other categories, one point for a 'yes', and half for a 'sometimes' and no points for a 'no' answer.

Analysis of replies

You now have three figures based on the answers to the three questionnaires. If there is an obvious and marked difference between them, so that one stands out as being far more 'you' than any of the others (a difference of two points or more) then that is your dominant characteristic.

Any combination of results is however possible, and there is no 'right' or 'wrong' mix of glandular types that is better than any other. You are what you are. But, your type may slowly alter. There are many cases of individuals who are one combination of types at the outset and who slowly alter to another. This can happen if, at the beginning, your characteristics are dominated by over-or under-function of one of the hormonal factors which we are using as a guide to your individuality. After sometime on a diet tailored to meet those needs, together with the particular supplements that are indicated this can resolve itself and a new pattern of glandular (or hormonal) function may appear.

It is therefore suggested that you repeat the assessment after 9 to 12 months and alter the dietary pattern accordingly, if there has been a marked alteration. The likelihood of a change in pattern is greater the worse your current general level of health is.

If there is no great difference between the results of the assessments (questionnaires), thyroid four, pituitary three and adrenal four or some such pattern, then it is unlikely that you have any particular dominant endocrine aspect and you can be considered as a 'mixed' type. The compiler of one method of body assessment, Dr Sheldon, stated the truism that the individual will always defy statistics. But, whilst many of us are a combination of three types, there is usually a dominant one. The obvious physical characteristics of the three categories may help to pin down the assessment more exactly.

Thyroid dominant type (thyroid assessment marks scored higher than the other types) is usually identifiable by having all, or some, of the following outstanding features: delicate or fine features; little body hair; head-hair silky; large, prominent eyes; graceful neck; small teeth not particularly resistant to decay; body contours mainly long and unusually thin; hands and fingers graceful. Generally characterized as 'highly strung'. Females tend to have short menstrual cycles (14-21) days.

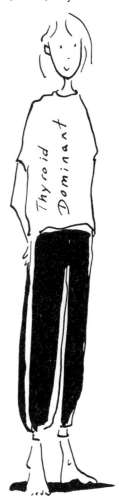

The pituitary dominant individual is characterized by all, or some, of the following features: large head, high domes and often a prominent forehead; joints tend to be lax and over-mobile; moons of fingers tend to be well-developed; teeth are unusually large, particularly the incisors.

The adrenal dominant individual is usually possessed of a number of the following characteristics: curly hair; low hair line; large teeth, extremely resistant to decay; heavy jaw; dry, warm skin; short neck; broad chest; protuberant abdomen; thick or short fingers and toes. In general this person is more like a draught horse than a racehorse!

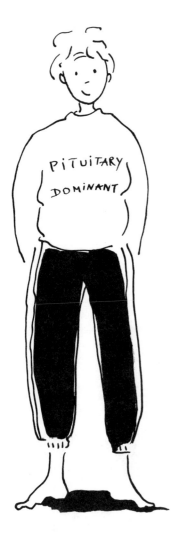
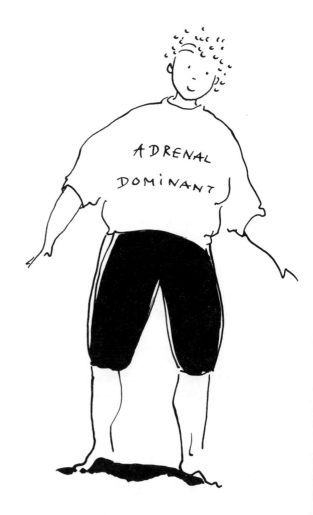

You should now have some essential information upon which we can work. If your dominant glandular feature is pituitary then, within broad limits, your ideal dietary pattern is that of a vegetarian. Animal protein should therefore play only a limited role in your dietary pattern. If your dominant glandular feature indicates you to be thyroid type, then your diet should contain a good mix of desirable foods neither totally vegetarian nor excessively meat-orientated. If you have emerged from the assessment as an adrenal type then your diet should contain a high level of animal protein and very little starchy or sugary food. More specific dietary suggestions for the different types will be given later.

The underarm test and the blood-pressure test can be high or low (over- or underactive thyroid or underactive adrenals) irrespective of what type you are. The result of these tests will determine whether or not you need particular nutritional supplementation. These tests should be reassessed after three to six months to see if thyroid and/or adrenal function has tended towards normal.

If you begin to follow the dietary patterns indicated by your particular hormonal 'type' and follow the advice relating to the thyroid and adrenal test results, then you will revolutionize your metabolism and at last be eating according to the particular needs of your body. The results of this should be rapidly evident, in terms of improved health and a weight pattern that is right for you. The following chapters will deal with the particular need of each type as well as the individual needs indicated by the thyroid and adrenal tests.

If there is no clear cut difference in your test results (one type at least two points more than the others) then use the general indications of characterisitcs to see which you most closely resemble. In this way you should be able to identify your closest approximation of a type in order to know what dietary pattern to follow. If no clear distinction emerges then stay on the basic diet already described.

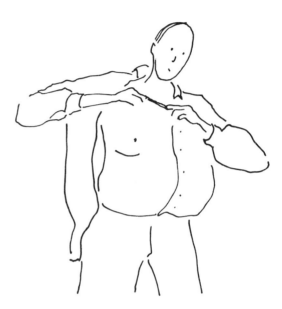

There are two further tests which can be used to add force to the above information. These are designed to show whether your metabolism is best suited to a vegetarian or a meat eating mode. They are not foolproof but do, in the majority of cases, confirm what we have deduced from the assessments as discussed above.

These two tests are subjective, in that they rely upon your own judgement as to how you feel, and so should not be used independently of the questionnaire assessments. They are meant to confirm your results and in most cases, they will. If they contradict them it may be that you have not answered the questions as accurately as you might, or that you are a 'borderline' between two 'types', and that you are therefore best suited to a mixed feeding pattern rather than a vegetarian or high protein extreme.

Confirmation test 1

From a health food store obtain a bottle of niacin or nicotinic acid tablets (not nicotinamide). On waking, and on an empty stomach, take 50 milligrams of niacin. Within half an hour your skin, and especially your face, may become reddened (like a hot flush) and you may feel very hot and itchy. If this happens then you are probably an adrenal type and your diet should contain a fairly high proportion of meat and animal protein.

If you simply feel warmer within half an hour, but do not actually glow or feel hot and itchy, then you are a balanced mixed-diet feeder (thyroid type). If you feel no change whatever then you are a predominantly vegetarian feeder.

The results thus obtained and by taking 50 mgms of niacin (Vitamin B_3) on an empty stomach can be confirmed by doing the test again later (on another day—always on an empty stomach), or by doing the following test:

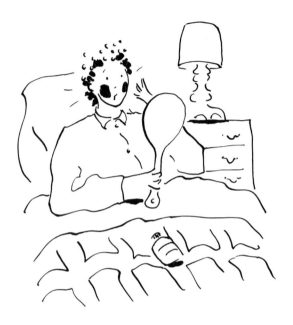

Confirmation test 2

From a chemist, or health store, obtain vitamin C (ascorbic acid) in one gram capsules, or tablets and, each day for three days, take eight grams (spread the intake throughout the day, do not take them all at once). You may find that your bowels become loose. You can disregard this as it will pass after you stop the high vitamin C intake. If, during the period of high C intake you feel depressed, lethargic, tired and edgy (or, in the case of women, if you develop vaginal irritation), then this confirms you as an adrenal-dominant meat-eater.

If you notice no particular change at all then you are probably a mixed-feeder (thyroid type) but if you become energetic, sleep better and generally feel better than average, then you are probably a pituitary-dominant, vegetarian-inclined feeder.

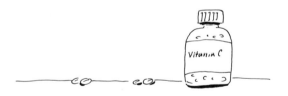

As I have said, these tests (based on Dr William Kelley's work) are not claimed to be infallible, but they can be used as guidelines and to confirm your assessment results before you embark on the changes in eating pattern suggested in the following chapters.

Diet for your metabolic type

How is any individual to know which diet suits him best, without trying them all and then comparing? One way, of course, is to identify your needs and to meet them. This is our current task, which I believe to be more direct than wading through several hundred variations on the theme of a slimming programme.

If you have answered the questions in the previous chapter then you should at least have an awareness of the variations that exist between the thyroid, pituitary and adrenal types.

The first important point to establish is that we are all combinations of all the three types. It may be that one obviously dominates your particular make-up, but it is in their ratios, one to another, that we will see the subtle individual aspects that make you unique. Compare your results, and note which has scored highest (if any).

This is your dominant glandular metabolic type. Compare it with the notes in this chapter, which describe in more detail the characteristics of that type, and also the other types, and decide whether indeed the descriptions, *in the main*, are true for you. If not, and if you do the questionnaires again and are still not able to identify yourself clearly, it is probable that you are a well-mixed and well-balanced type, and the basic dietary pattern outlined on pages 31-33 should suit you adequately.

If, after due consideration of the expanded descriptions in this chapter, as well as the questionnaire results, you are able to identify yourself as a particular type, then proceed to the dietary pattern which is outlined for that type in Chapter 8 and begin, over the coming weeks, to introduce that pattern of eating. It is not something to rush at, indeed it should take some time for

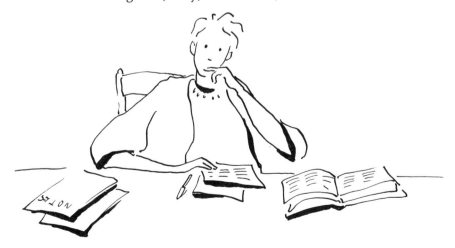

you to adjust to. As long as a month can be taken in transition. This diet is your correct metabolic one, and provides you with the balance of foods which your particular physiological make-up is best able to digest, and derive nutrients from. Of course it may require adjustment if it is very different from the pattern that you previously followed.

Also, at this stage, begin to incorporate the special nutrients which your type needs. This is not a long term necessity, but should be followed for six months at least. Remember that there will be some nutrients (supplements of nutritional factors) which you should take as part of the transition to your new pattern of eating.

There is also a probability, unless you are extraordinarily well balanced nutritionally and metabolically speaking that, when you have completed the nutritional assessment questionnaires in the following chapters, you will begin to meet those unique requirements that we have discussed previously. These will depend, as you will see when you begin to go through the questionnaires, on very individual characteristics. It may seem to you that supplements should not be necessary if the diet is right. Because of a variety of factors, including modern agricultural and marketing methods, our food contains less than it ought of the substances we are concerned with, in this regard: the minerals, trace elements and vitamins.

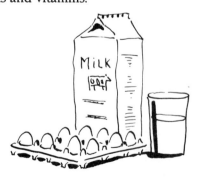

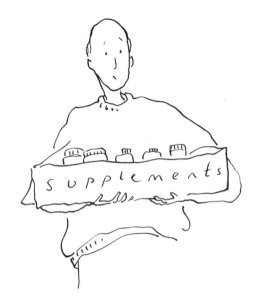

It is also a proven fact that such substances as manganese, for example, are largely deficient in Western man, and to replace in the body the amounts that are necessary to improve function (manganese has a great deal to do with glucose and fat metabolism, so you can see how important it is to our cause) requires up to six months of regular supplementation. It would take years to try to do the same thing by diet alone. This example is meant to help you put aside doubts you may have about taking supplements.

We will be suggesting only those that your honest appraisal of yourself indicates as essential, and only in quantities that are acceptable. I cannot stress strongly enough how important this aspect of the programme is to the achievement of your goal of optimum health and weight. Ultimately, it will be necessary for you to reassess yourself by re-doing the questionnaires, and you will be amazed to find that you will require less and less supplementation as you approach the ideal standard of weight and health that you can expect.

The thyroid type

This person, when in good health, is usually of delicate physical construction, with a thin body, long chest and neck, and finely-made hands with shapely fingers. The hair is usually fine or silky, and there is little body hair apart from the underarms and the genital area. The eyes are usually large, perhaps prominent, and expressive. The thyroid individual has moderately small, narrowly-spaced teeth which are not particularly well protected from caries. The arch of the palate is high, rather than low. The thyroid type has heightened sensitivity of the sexual organs, and indeed the whole state of the nervous system is sensitive and quickly aroused. Bieler, in his books, talks of this type being the 'race-horse' type, rather than the draught horse—which could be said to characterize some aspects of the adrenal type.

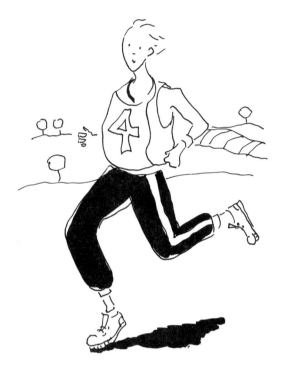

Unless there are accompanying hormonal difficulties the thyroid type is unlikely to have weight problems, because of the rapid oxidation and metabolic activity characteristic of the type. The character of the thyroid type is sometimes said to be one which is easily dissatisfied (with environment, job, relationships, etc). Concentration is often difficult, and fatigue common. Menstruation may take place at shorter intervals than average, sometimes as often as fortnightly. Insomnia and restlessness are frequently symptoms, and dreams are likely to be unpleasant. Normally, the thyroid type wakes early and is refreshed.

The dietary pattern of the thyroid type is one in which a balanced mixed diet is needed, without excessive amounts of animal protein. As a rule the thyroid individual's metabolism is fast (although there may be exceptions, as you will note from doing the underarm temperature tests, as well as by answering some of the questions in the next chapter). As a result of this, more overall care is called for in the selection of food. As a guideline, salt should play only a small part in the thyroid type's diet and calcium-rich foods are more important than in the other types.

It is often preferable, because of the particular metabolic factors operating in this type, to eat a number of small meals daily, rather than three set meals. A pattern of five or six snack meals is probably suitable. The thyroid type is often healthier and happier if meat is in little evidence in the diet, with proteins such as fish, seafood and perhaps poultry, taking its place. This type should be particularly careful about 'hidden' salt in foods such as cheese, and processed foods of all sorts. The dietary pattern, as outlined on pages 31-33 and which you should by now be following, therefore requires the following modifications if you are a thyroid dominant type:

Thyroid type menu

Breakfast: Wholegrain and seed dish, plus natural yogurt *or* buttermilk, or skim milk. *Or*, on alternate days one egg, (not fried). One slice wholemeal bread or toast and a scraping of butter. *Or* soaked dried fruit and seeds (sunflower, pumpkin, sesame, etc.) Herb tea, coffee substitute or unsweetened fruit juice.

Mid morning: Fresh fruit (apple, banana, pear etc.). *Or* handful of seeds (as above).

Lunch: Seafood and salad; *or* seafood and cooked fresh green vegetables. *Or* cereal/pulse dish and salad.

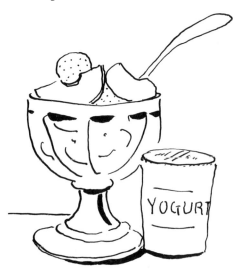

Mid-afternoon: Natural yogurt *or* fresh fruit *or* seeds.

Evening meal: Poultry *or* fish served with fresh vegetables, raw or cooked or a combination of both. Plus brown rice *or* potato salad.

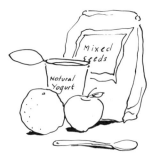

Food notes

If a vegetarian combination (pulse cereal) is eaten at one main meal then fish or poultry can be eaten at the other. The vegetarian meal can be served either as lunch or as dinner.

All meals should be moderate, not containing more than one course, and quantities should match appetite. Quantities are not given since, by sticking to wholefoods and frequent snack-type meals, the thyroid type will adjust to smallish helpings.

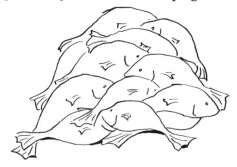

Salt should be strictly limited, and saltless cooking adopted if at all possible. Note that all cheese, including cottage cheese, is high in salt. The thyroid type needs additional supplies of calcium so the use of milk products, such as yogurt, is desirable. A certain increase in complex carbohydrates, such as wholemeal bread, brown rice, and all root vegetables, fruits and seeds, is highly desirable. The brassica family of vegetables which includes cabbage, cauliflower and broccoli is highly beneficial for this type.

Supplements for the thyroid type

Kelp, 1g

Dolomite (calcium and magnesium) 3 tablets.

Continue with brewer's yeast (9 tablets daily) until the completion of the questionnaires in subsequent chapters, when more specific indications of supplements may be indicated.

All these supplements should be taken with meals.

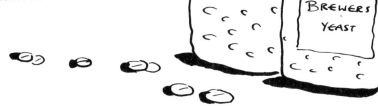

Exercise for the thyroid type

The type of exercise programme required by the three types may also vary. To a large extent this will be determined by the use of the principles explained in relation to achieving your optimum pulse rate. However, it is worth emphasizing that the type of exercise undertaken will also influence the success of the programme.

The thyroid type is better avoiding competitive exercise patterns and should, as with meals, do little and often, rather than trying to do too much at one time.

Walking, cycling and swimming are ideal exercises for the thyroid type, and morning is probably the best time for these pursuits. Exercises to be carried out at home are in the next section, together with relaxation and imagery techniques.

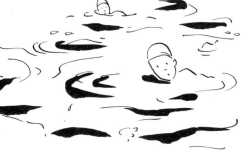

The pituitary type

The typical pituitary type is most often fairly tall, with long extremities, long fingers, and a large head. The forehead is frequently very prominent, as are the bones above the eyes, making the eyebrows a strong feature. The upper lip is usually longer than average, and this often leads to the pituitary man growing a moustache. The pituitary person has larger than average teeth, notably the ones in the front, such as the incisors.

A characteristic of this type is that the ligaments which bind the joints are often on the lax side, and this can lead to such problems as flat feet or knock knees being manifest. One unusual pointer that has been noted in the pituitary type is that the moons on the finger nails are particularly noticeable and well formed. The knuckles of the hands often appear larger than normal, leading to difficulty in wearing rings.

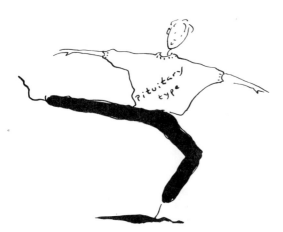

This person is often strongly intuitive with a creative or artistic drive and temperament. These people tolerate pain well, but, whilst they have good digestion if eating the foods that are designed for their needs they suffer from a slightly greater degree of illness than average. Their sexual drive is very strong.

Pituitary type menu

Breakfast: Muesli (cereals, nuts and seeds) with fresh and dried fruit. Natural yogurt. *Or* wholemeal bread (or toast) and an egg (4 to 5 weekly). Fruit. Drink herb tea or coffee substitute or unsweetened fruit juice.

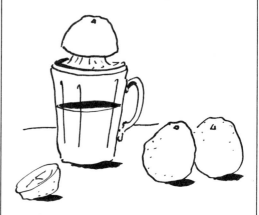

Lunch: Mixed raw or cooked salad plus millet *or* rice savoury, and seeds and nuts *or* jacket potato. Dress salad with pure vegetable oil and lemon juice.

Evening meal: Fish *or* chicken *or* vegetarian savoury and fresh vegetables, raw or cooked. Once a week have a raw food day on which you eat nothing but fruits, cereals, seeds, nuts and salads. Eat as much of these as you wish.

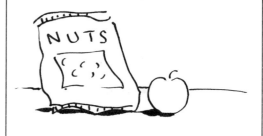

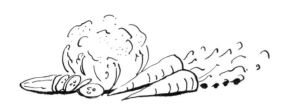

Food notes

From the dietary viewpoint these people are even more strongly advised to avoid salt than the thyroid type. In fact they often have a strong dislike of salted foods. The emphasis in the dietary pattern is on vegetables and plant products as a whole, including fruits, nuts, grains, pulses and seeds. This is the group that often do well as vegetarians and, usually, do best on a diet low in animal protein.

The pattern of eating should therefore include, for breakfast, a mixture of seeds and nuts and grains (muesli) which can be bought (no sugar, please, so check the label) or made yourself, by buying the ingredients separately and fruit, both fresh and dried.

One of the main meals should be a salad, as in the basic diet outlined on page 31, but without animal protein and with the addition of seeds (sunflower, pumpkin, etc.) and nuts, as well as rice or millet savoury (see the recipe section). The other main meal should of course emphasize the protein needs of the body but in this case, this need not necessarily be from red meat sources.

Eggs can be eaten (four or five a week is adequate) as can other forms of animal protein, such as a little fish or chicken. Cheese should be avoided, because of its salt content. The choice as to whether to eat animal protein depends upon your inner feelings. It is true to say that most pituitary types do well on a vegetarian dietary pattern, but this may not be suitable from a social or practical viewpoint. If you are going to opt for a no meat, no fish, diet, then you will need to learn how you can maintain health and energy levels from vegetable sources alone by the judicious combining of certain different families of foods, thus giving your body its requirements of protein and general nutrients.

The protein meal in the pituitary type's menu, then, might be of vegetarian or animal protein. Even if it is the latter, it should contain a good sized plate of fresh vegetables or salad to accompany the protein dish. Fruit should be eaten as a dessert and as snacks.

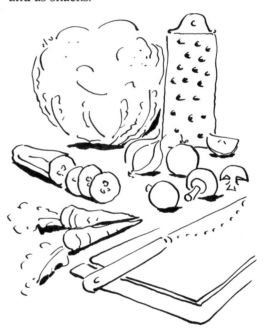

Once a week pituitary people should give themselves a 'raw food' day, in which they eat salads and fruit only, without anything cooked. On this day the protein intake will be derived from mixing seeds, nuts and grains, as in the muesli mix. There exists a tendency for the pituitary type to lean heavily on the use of stimulants, such as coffee, tea or alcohol. This must be controlled and the appropriate diet and supplements will assist in this.

Supplements for the pituitary type

Zinc, 25mg (as B_{13} — zinc also called zinc orotate),

Lecithin, 1000mg

Vitamin B_6 (pyridoxine), 25mg

Brewer's yeast, 9 tablets daily

All to be taken with food.

In contrast to the thyroid type no snacks should be eaten between meals by the pituitary type. Quantities should be dictated by appetite. As the bulk of the food suggested is of a complex carboydrate, or high fibre, type, it is very difficult to overeat on this type of diet. The exercise programme will assist in this aspect of things as well.

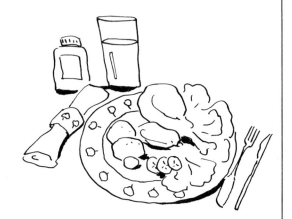

Exercise for the pituitary type

The exercise pattern of the pituitary type should involve such slow and stretching activities as yoga or tai chi chuan, as well as regular walks and non-violent pursuits such as swimming and cycling.

Exercise will be found in the next section, together with relaxation and guided imagery methods.

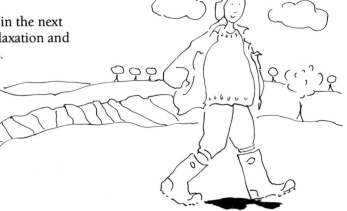

The adrenal type

The adrenal type could not be more different from the pituitary. This is the person with large, often coarse features and a lot of body and head hair, which is often curly. The hairline is usually quite low, giving the appearance of a less developed forehead, than the other types. The nose tends to be large with prominent nostrils. The teeth are large and strong, very resistant to decay. The lips are well coloured as a result of the excellent circulation that the adrenal type possesses. The palate, like the other features, is wide and low. The facial characteristics are often dominated by a strong lower jaw, and the head as a whole is wide and solid. The ears, and especially the lobes, are large and fleshy. The neck is short—bulldog-like describes the adrenal type well. The skin is warm to the touch, and this type seldom complains of the cold.

The abdomen may be protruding, and the extremities may be short and thick, as might the fingers. In contrast to the pituitary type, the moons on the nails are small or absent.

One of the characteristics of true adrenal types is their energy, which is almost inexhaustible. The digestive system is extremely strong, which enables this type to eat almost anything without apparent ill effects.

This type has strong muscular tone; rapid bowel evacuations (seldom constipated) and is very resistant to bacterial infection.

In character he is easy going and good natured. Sleep is never a problem, and his gregarious qualities, along with his natural energy and good nature, give him a large circle of friends. The intelligence level of this type is usually slightly lower than the others, on average.

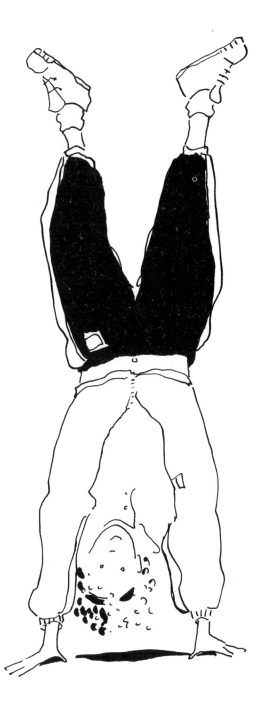

Adrenal type menu

Breakfast: Should include some animal protein, in the form of eggs (six to seven weekly) *or* fish, as well as a cereal such as muesli *or* oatmeal porridge with buttermilk *or* skim milk, *or* yogurt; and wholemeal toast and a scraping of butter. An item of fruit may also be added. Drink herb tea or coffee substitute.

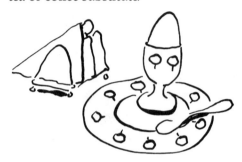

Lunch: Should include three to five ounces of lean meat, *or* fish, *or* poultry (skinned), and a large mixed or green salad, and/or a large plate of cooked vegetables. Fresh fruit for dessert.

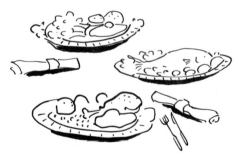

Evening meal: Should have a similar pattern except that if meat was eaten at lunch then fish should be eaten now, and vice-versa, again with salad or fresh cooked vegetables. The quantities of animal protein should not exceed 10 oz (300g) a day, and a little less would be better.

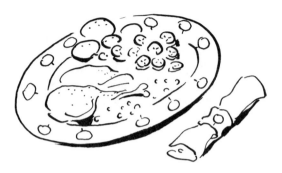

Food notes

Nutritionally, this type requires a high protein diet and, since digestion and elimination are excellent, they can cope with this without too much difficulty. Three good-sized meals daily are the diet, with breakfast a feature of this pattern. The pattern should differ from the basic diet, as outlined on pages 31-33 as follows:

The danger inherent in such a diet, even for adrenal types, is that the fat content of the protein will cause damage, so this aspect requires close watching. Avoid the fat contained in muscle meat (steak etc.) and concentrate instead on organ meat (liver etc.), fish, and poultry (avoiding the skin). These are guidelines wich can result in a marked reduction in fat intake. Frying should be avoided.

It is also desirable that the excellent appetite be employed to include in the diet as much salad and fruit as is possible, to help counteract the long term nutrient imbalance that can result from a high protein diet. It is advisable for adrenal types to minimize the use of carbohydrates such as bread, pasta, etc., as this can allow for excessive weight gains. Any snacks (and these should be avoided if possible) should be of fresh fruit. No *additional* carbohydrate should be eaten (no bread, pasta, etc.).

Supplements for the adrenal type

Wheatgerm, at least 1 tablespoon daily

Vitamin B_6, 50mg

Garlic capsules, 3 daily

Selenium, 50 mcg

Brewer's yeast, 9 tablets per day

All these to be taken with meals (the wheatgerm can be sprinkled on salad or cereal food).

Exercise for the adrenal type

The exercise pattern of this type requires that an element of competitive drive be included, if possible. In any case, the pattern should include more rapid forms of exercise than the other types.

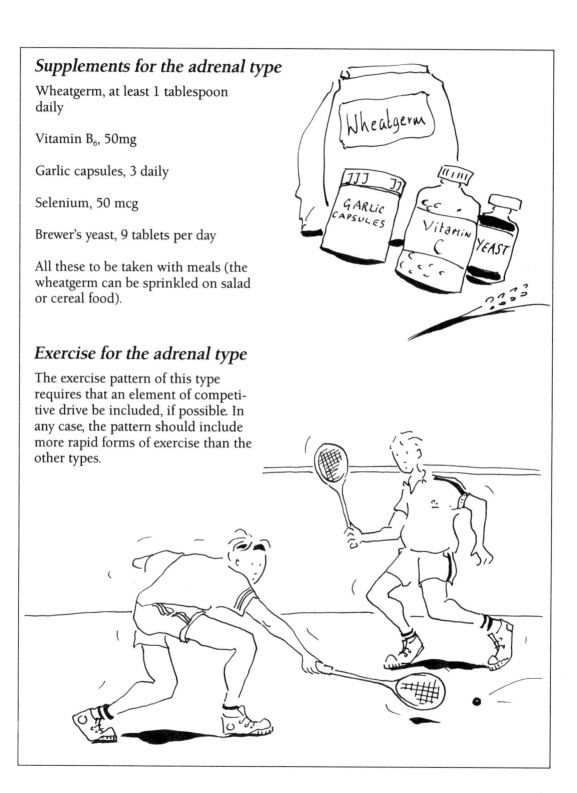

Dietary summary

Thyroid type: Fish and poultry instead of meat. Cut out salt. No cheese; add skimmed milk and/or buttermilk to breakfast, otherwise stick to basic dietary pattern. Eat several small meals, rather than large ones.

Daily supplements: 1g kelp. 3 Dolomite (calcium & magnesium) tablets. 9 brewer's yeast tablets.

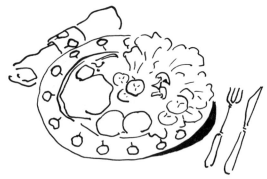

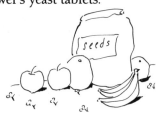

Pituitary type: No salt. No meat. Additional salad, fruit and grains, seeds and nuts, to replace animal protein. Some fish and poultry if desired. Raw food day, weekly. Care required regarding tendency to use of stimulants such as coffee, alcohol and sugar-rich foods.

Daily supplements: 1000mg Lecithin. 9 brewer's yeast tablets. 25mg zinc. 25mg vitamin B_6.

Brewer's yeast

The advice regarding the taking of brewer's yeast should be ignored if you have had a history of Candida infections (thrush) or if you are particularly prone to depression, abdominal bloating, cystitis or vaginal discharges. If these symptoms are current, and persistent you may be suffering from a Candida infection (Candida is a form of yeast that lives in all of us). This could have been aggravated by a course of antibiotics, the contraceptive pill, or stress factors. In any case, the dietary pattern we have outlined in the book will help, but it is well to avoid yeast-containing foods. Also add to your diet the taking of Acidophilus powder (this is a bacteria which makes yogurt for us, from milk, and which helps to control Candida). Take 1g daily. A high potency acidophilus powder (Superdophilus) can be obtained from G&G Supplies, listed on page 118.

This powder can be obtained from suppliers listed at the end of this book. Also take 300mcg Biotin (a B vitamin) after each meal and 2 tablespoons of olive oil daily (for its oleic acid content). Eat as much raw garlic as you can.

If brewer's yeast is not contraindicated, because of the possibility of a Candida infection then continue to take it until the completion of the questionnaires in subsequent chapters, which will indicate whether or not there is a need for its continued use.

Adrenal type: Increase animal protein (one meat meal and one fish or poultry meal daily). Less 'muscle' meat, and more organ meats desirable. Watch fat intake. Increase salads to balance animal protein intake. Three large meals daily. It is necessary to watch carbohydrate intake if weight problems are to be avoided.

Daily supplements: 1 tablespoon wheatgerm. 50mg vitamin B_6. 3 garlic capsules. 50mcg selenium. 9 brewer's yeast tablets.

'Mixed' or undefined type: Stick to basic diet. (Chapter 3, pages 31-33) and take 9 brewer's yeast tablets daily with food (3 per meal).

Weight problems analysed by type

The thyroid type is unlikely to have weight problems. This is true, unless the gland becomes underactive, and this can be assessed in the questionnaire section (Chapters 8 and 9) as well as by the underarm temperature test.

The pituitary type is the person who gathers weight either from the waist upwards only, or the waist downwards only. This type is a tallish individual: the female is often described as 'horsey'. They may have slim legs and arms, and be well proportioned above the waist, with large hips and buttocks; or, conversely, have a reasonably well-proportioned waist and lower half, and be heavy across the chest and shoulder area.

The adrenal type is the one who least conforms with the current ideal dimensions laid down by fashion. This is the person who may, by the time they are approaching their mid-thirties, have lost the definition between bust and hips. In other words, the waistline spreads so that there exists a barrel-like silhouette. Since the adrenal type is shorter than the others, on average, and since the bone structure and muscular development is of the heavy type, it is fair to say that there is no possibility of this type conforming to the popular 'model' image.

If the adrenal type follows the diet outlined, together with the supplements recommended, as well as the exercise pattern, they will adjust to their optimum level of weight. This may well be a level which is as much as 11 to 15 pounds (5 to 7 kilos) above the weight-for-height figure commonly taken as the ideal. I would urge the adrenal person to accept that this is the ideal weight for them, and not to employ energy and effort towards an impossible dream.

The pituitary individual will find that the areas of additional weight they have acquired can be trimmed by the judicious application of the dietary measures and exercises, although the areas on which they have accumulated extra fat will still have the tendency to enlarge if dietary indiscretions recur.

The thyroid type is often underweight, (especially if the thyroid is a little overactive). However, they may be overweight, in a puffy, sluggish manner if the thyroid is underfunctioning, and this actually requires a degree of special consideration, which we will discuss after the questionnaire section.

It is possible for any of the types discussed to have an under or overfunctioning thyroid, and an under or overactive adrenal function. You will have indi-

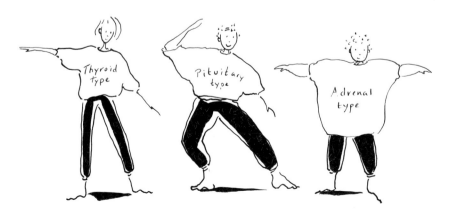

cations of this as a result of the underarm temperature and blood-pressure tests described in Chapter 4.

There are particular glandular and other nutrient supplements which will be suggested, depending upon these and the questionnaire results and this advice will be given after the endocrine appraisal questions have been answered (Chapter 8). Our next immediate task will be to give particular exercise, and guided imagery patterns for the three basic types that have been discussed so far.

So far so good

You should by this stage have altered your diet, along the lines suggested in the opening chapters of the book. You should have abandoned, or modified, your intake of the 'tasty toxins', that we discussed in detail. You should have begun to do simple stretching exercises. You should be aware of the use of your pulse as a guide to your ideal rate of achievement during the active exercise which you should have begun in a simple, but regular, manner.

Now having identified your place in the range of 'types' you should, if you are reasonably sure where you fit in, begin to alter the pattern of eating to that suggested for your particular type. The supplements that go with that identification should be included in your new programme. As before, take your time in making changes. Do one thing at a time so that, over a period of a month or so, you reach the pattern as outlined.

If you are still not clear as to which of the types you are, then stick with the basic diet as outlined in Chapter 2. This is a balanced, health-promoting diet which only requires modifying if there are clear indications as to your being a particular type. If you do not fit into a particular mould and you consider yourself to be overweight, then chances are your additional weight is the result of factors which we will assist in correcting when we have completed the health assessment section and you have adopted the suggestions that accompany it.

If you cannot be slotted into a particular type, then the chances of achieving healthy weight reduction are actually higher than if you are a clear adrenal or pituitary type. As I have pointed out, it is often normal for these types to be above average weight. This does not mean that they are above their normal weight, but only that they are above an average which bears no relation to their own particular metabolic and physiological type.

Our aim is health. If your weight is above *your* normal, then good health will bring a weight adjustment towards that norm. If *your* normal is to be an above average weight, then health will not bring much weight change. Whatever happens, by following the advice which you are patiently gathering together to fit your own needs, you will produce a trend towards a higher level of health and good function which will more than amply reward your efforts.

General advice

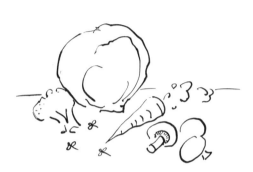

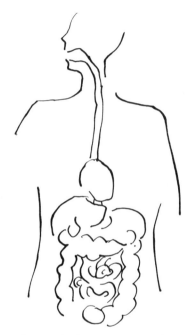

Vegetarianism

Since it has been suggested that it is desirable for some individuals to tend towards a vegetarian mode of eating and that all 'types' can benefit from a vegetarian meal as part of their normal pattern, it is as well to discuss this way of eating briefly.

There are inherent benefits to be derived from a vegetarian diet. It is clear that a balanced diet which eliminates animal protein confers advantages in terms of health. There is statistically less chance of developing cancer, coronary disease, high blood-pressure, and a multitude of other less dramatic ailments, by virtue of being a vegetarian.

It has been argued that, by looking at man's physiological structure, it is apparent that we are designed for a vegetarian lifestyle. Everything, from our teeth to our digestive system, our pores to our method of consuming water, points to this.

It is also argued that over the many thousands of years of adaptation to a mixed diet (i.e., one that includes meat) man has evolved into a variety of patterns of eating, all of which are ideal for him. There is therefore no single diet ideal for everyone. To some extent we have covered this in our attempt to define your particular requirements as far as food is concerned.

It may be that, whilst the original blueprint called for humanity to be vegetarian, this is no longer the case for all people. If you are a natural vegetarian, and if you wish to succeed in providing your body with adequate nutrients to maintain health, then it is essential for you to understand that, with a little planning, you can achieve both an exciting dietary pattern and excellent health.

Protein is made up of substances called amino acids. When animal protein is consumed the eater is taking advantage of the animal's effort at synthesizing 'complete' protein from plant sources. When a vegetarian attempts to provide his body with complete protein from plant sources, he has to combine amino acids, which are present in different plant foods in varying ratios, in such a way as to provide his body with the wherewithal to make its own complete protein.

Thus, the combining of cereals (wheat, rice, millet, barley, oats and rye) with a pulse, such as lentils, chick peas (garbanzos) or butter (lima) beans, will give just such an ideal mixture.

Of course, since the majority of vegetarians continue eating eggs and dairy products, they are getting complete proteins as well. It is only when these are also jettisoned, and the vegetarian becomes a vegan, that infinite care is required to ensure the intake of balanced protein combinations from plants.

In the advice given here no such extreme is recommended. Indeed, in the vegetarian-style diet suggested for pituitary types, who are best suited to this dietary pattern, the recommendations incorporate some fish or poultry, if desired, and the adoption of a no flesh, no fish pattern is optional.

So the need for constant attention to such combinations of cereals and pulses may appear unnecessary. But it is important for good health to maintain a steady supply of protein and, even if animal protein is being avoided only on alternate days, it is necessary to ensure that on these days a sound vegetable protein meal is eaten. The vegetarian can enjoy a wide variety of foods and, indeed, often has a more adventurous time foodwise than someone who follows a routine of meat and vegetables on a daily basis.

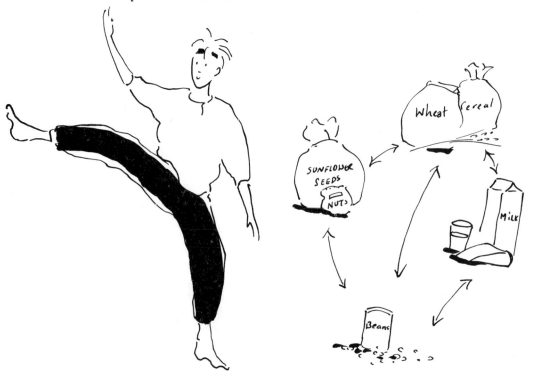

Raw foods

One of the most important elements of any dietary pattern that is aiming to provide us with our basic needs is the provision in it of adequate amounts of raw food. Fresh salad and vegetables of all sorts, as well as fruits, are a vital source of vitamins and minerals, and are also well stocked with fibre, which is so vital for health. Whichever type you are, I would urge you to get into the habit of eating raw food at each meal, and of having side salads and main salads as often as possible.

If at any time you just want to gorge yourself, try doing it on a crunchy salad. Chew each mouthful well and you will stop eating far sooner than on any other type of food.

Salads should include as wide a mixture of fresh ingredients as are available. Everything from dandelion leaves to raw cauliflower and mushrooms can be included. I have listed some of the vegetables that can be eaten raw in the salad recipes given later, and would urge you to think of a salad as an adventure in terms of its range of textures, colours, flavours and odours.

A well prepared salad, in which the ingredients have been chopped, shredded, sliced and mixed, and dressed appropriately (no salt, no vinegar) becomes the centrepiece of a meal. There is always something new in season, and the new experiences in taste and enjoyment that can be derived from salads alone will amaze you.

Accompany with a jacket potato, a brown rice dish or wholemeal bread, along with a sprinkling of seeds such as sunflower, pumpkin or sesame, and you have a feast.

It is worth urging all who approach the task of making such meals interesting to learn the simple art of sprouting seeds for salads. Such flavours as alfalfa and fenugreek, when added to salads, are sheer delight. The nutritive value of sprouted seeds is enormous and they come as close as modern man can get to being purely organic, since all you add to them is water and then wait for them to sprout. Freshness, cleanliness and imagination are all that it takes to construct a salad meal, which can be as enjoyable in midwinter as midsummer.

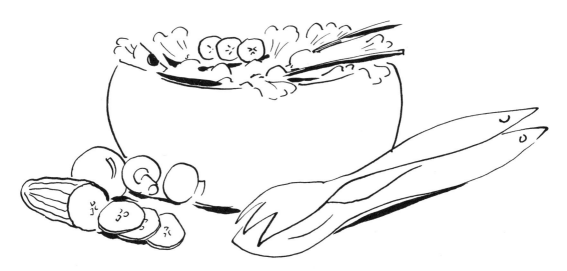

Salad ingredients

The mixing together of a selection of raw vegetables is one definition of a salad. In this regard, all of the following can be eaten raw in salads. The greater the variety the greater the degree of interest and the more pleasure and nutrient value there will be.

Carrots; lettuce; cucumber; tomatoes; artichoke; dandelion; sprouted seeds; fennel; kale, chives; chicory; white and red cabbage; radish; avocado; mustard and cress; nasturtium leaves; mushrooms; leeks; broccoli; peppers; cauliflower; green peas; parsley; mint; endive; turnips; garlic; kohl rabi; watercress; spinach; green beans; Brussels sprouts; parsnips; beetroot, etc.

All root vegetables, such as raw beetroot and carrot, should be prepared by grating them on the finest part of the grater as close to meal time as possible to avoid undue nutrient loss through oxidation.

A few drops of lemon juice may be added (for example) to grated carrot or grated raw beetroot (beet).

Use herbs such as mint, garlic and parsley generously to enhance salads and heighten flavours.

A selection of any five or six items on the list above should be decoratively arranged so that there is a contrast of colours and textures. The sight of an all-green salad is lightened and made more exciting to the palate by the addition of a few touches of red (radish, red pepper) or orange (carrot).

One grated raw vegetable, some coleslaw mixture plus one or two green salad vegetables (watercress, chicory) and sprinkling of seeds and nuts, as well as some sprouting seeds (mung beans, alfalfa) plus a light dressing (which can include olive oil, lemon juice, crushed garlic, yogurt) and/or the addition of herbs such as mint or parsley, will present the taste senses with a feast of flavours.

There is no end to the variety available. Depending upon seasonal changes and economic factors salads are always possible and should always be interesting and enjoyable.

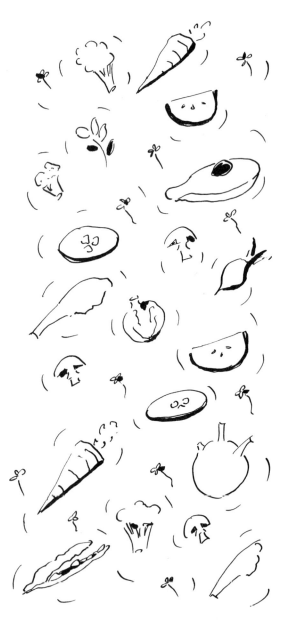

Simple rules

The use of anything refined, or canned, or preserved, or containing anything in the way of colouring or flavouring is not, in any way, a part of the pattern of eating that we are encouraging. Fresh, unprocessed and as natural as you can get, that is your aim.

Quantities are usually an essential part of any diet book. We have tried to keep such suggestions to a minimum. For one thing, few people actually abide by them, and for another it's my experience that, except in the most glaring of compulsive eater's, the provision of the pattern of eating that has been outlined will moderate, and modulate, the quantity of food eaten. In the case of people who find it hard to control their quantities (and these should pay extra attention to the tips in the previous section), by sticking to the guidelines of their 'type' and not stepping back into the world of 'tasty toxins' they will be able to achieve an improvement in health by virtue of the greater nutritional value of the food being eaten, as well as the fibre content.

Altogether, then, we have a pattern of reformed eating which approximates your unique requirements, as well as filling a particular need in so far as any weight or health problems are concered. All you have to do is to take one step at a time, and work your way towards the goals that we have outlined.

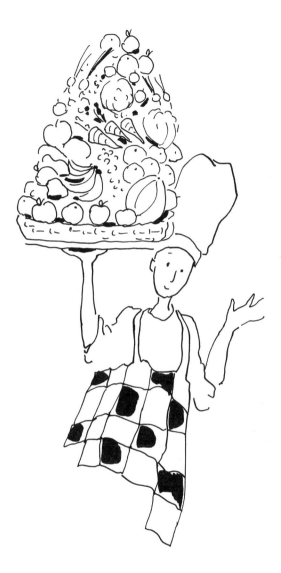

The following books are recommended. Some of them are bound to contain undesirable recipes, from our viewpoint. Watch out for any that include *cheese* or *fats*. These are not acceptable. No use should be allowed of white flour, white rice, or salt. You know how to replace these.

Avoid all cured, smoked, preserved, pickled, canned or dried meats or fishes (including sausages, bacon, hams).

Avoid all bottled sauces, dressings or pickles. Avoid anything containing salt or baking powders, unless these are salt-free. Avoid all food additives; soup or stock cubes; olives; margarine.

Learn to use herbs and spices in place of salt, and moderate amounts of potassium salt substitute.

Vegetable sautéing without fat or oil can be achieved by placing a little water in the bottom of a skillet or frying pan, adding the chopped vegetables and cooking until well done, over a moderate heat, stirring as needed. A little extra water can be added from time to time if the vegetables appear to be getting dry during the process. Another method is the placing of the chopped vegetables in a moderately hot non-stick pan, and cooking until done, stirring as required.

By avoiding fats and salted foods, and all refined carbohydrates, and by increasing your intake of wholefoods in line with your body type, you will reap rewards for your health and well-being out of all proportion to the small changes called for. As to alcohol, it is suggested that no more than the equivalent of one and a half glasses of wine be consumed daily. This is an absolute top limit, beyond which it is known that health hazards begin.

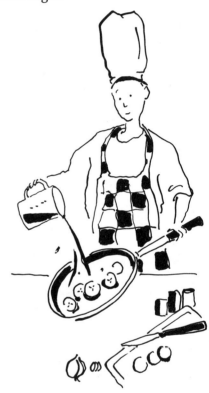

Book list

Pritikin Program for Diet and Exercise, Nathan Pritikin and Patrick McGrody, (Bantam Books 1981).
Your Personal Health Programme, Jeffrey Bland, (Thorsons, 1984).
Scott Ewing's Low Fat Luxury, Scott Ewing (Thorsons, 1988).
Food for Thought Cookbook, Guy Garrett and Kit Norman (Thorsons, 1987).
The Wharf Street Vegetarian Café Cookbook, Jill Gibbon (Thorsons, 1986).
No-Salt Cookery, Sarah Bounds, (Thorsons/NTP, 1984).
Wholegrain Recipe Book, Marlis Weber, (Thorsons, 1983).
Greek Vegetarian Cooking, Alkmini Chaitow, (Thorsons, 1982).

Advanced exercises

You should by now have been doing the introductory exercises as outlined in Chapter 3, for a month or so. This will have disciplined you to daily involvement in the three areas of exercise that are vital to total health:

- stretching,
- toning (sometimes described as aerobics),
- and relaxing.

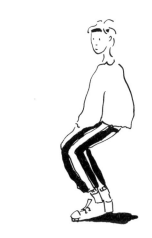

The stretching exercises are more important to some types than to others. If you are stiff-jointed they should be an integral part of your life, to prevent the slow seizing up of joints endured by so many people. They should precede your toning exercises, as part of the warm up.

Altogether they should take no more than *ten* minutes, as long as this is a daily pattern. If you are doing exercises only every other day (and you cannot do them less than this if you are to achieve your goals) then spend *twenty* minutes, preceding the toning exercises, on the stretching movements.

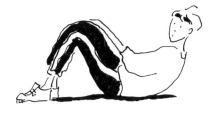

The toning, or aerobic, exercises are so important to your health and weight programme that I will emphasize this by repetition as we go along. After the toning session, several points will indicate that you have achieved your goal for the day. First, you will have done sufficient to raise, and maintain, your pulse rate at the level that you calculated previously. Second, you will almost certainly have had to do some heavy

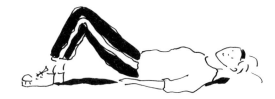

breathing, and you should have started perspiring.

The combination of deep, enforced breathing, sweating, and a raised pulse rate are your guides to successful, active exercise.

Your safety limit is within your control at all times, by virtue of monitoring your pulse rate. By the practise of taking your pulse, as you have gradually introduced the regular pattern of walking briskly each day (or at least every other day), you should by now be able to assess its level without having to count for a full minute.

This is of some importance, since you will not wish to interrupt your flow of your exercise by breaks of more than a few seconds. Count the pulse for ten seconds, and multiply by six to get a minute-rate. If you think that you might either not be getting near to your desired pulse rate, or, even more importantly, if you feel that you have exceeded your safe limit, then you must check thoroughly. Gradually you will have to do more to reach your desired level of pulse rate, as you become fitter and your circulatory and respiratory systems become tuned to the new demands that your programme is making on them. This is a marvellously encouraging process, because it is accompanied by a heightened sense of well-being and energy.

Have you considered that all this exercise is going to play havoc with your diet, as your appetite is going to be so stimulated that you might break away from your dietary pattern and binge and lose control? This is the exact opposite of what almost always happens. You find that by doing the exercise programme regularly (all three phases—stretching, toning and relaxation) your appetite will adjust to a far more desirable level than in the past when it may have tended to lead you astray. You will eat more sensibly and you will achieve a level of fitness you never thought possible by regularly doing these three phases of exercise.

The relaxation phase, which must conclude the pattern each time, will also include a visualization exercise, which you will find to be of immense value in unwinding and motivating you.

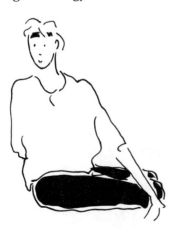

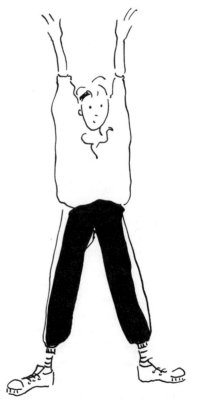

Stretching exercises

For all metabolic types: The only variation will be that your particular anatomical, and physiological state at the time will determine just how far you can get.

You will respond differently if you are a pituitary type (loose ligaments) than if you are an adrenal type (short, tight ligaments). So do not expect to achieve total degrees of stretch in all directions, even by repetition. What you are achieving is *your* best level of stretch, and this helps prepare the body for its other exercise tasks.

Once again start with the first movement, described in Chapter 3. Stand up straight with feet 15 inches (38 cm) apart, and hands clasped behind your back. Then allow yourself to bend forwards, from the hips, as far as is comfortable. Using no effort allow the weight of your body to stretch you forward, and down.

You should be aware of the backs of your legs being stretched tight. Hold the position for between one and two minutes, whilst you breathe deeply and slowly, allowing the stretch to achieve its maximum.

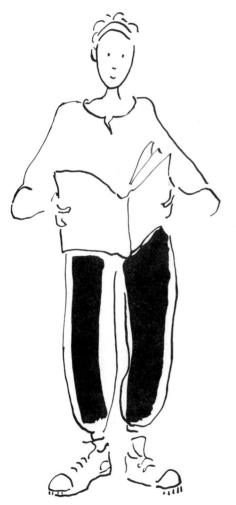

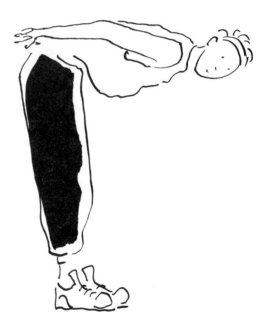

The next exercise in the stretching sequence is new. You may continue to use the introductory exercises, but you may also abandon them if you wish, in the interests of time, and follow these next movements instead.

Advanced stretch 1

Kneel on the floor with your knees together, and sit down on your feet. Your spine should be straight, and your hands should rest on your knees.

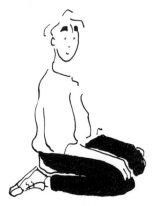

If this is not comfortable, then try sitting with your feet apart and your buttocks on a cushion between your legs.

If this in not uncomfortable see whether, at this stage, it is possible for you to separate your feet slightly to allow your buttocks to rest on the floor between your legs.

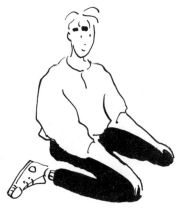

In time, the muscles of this area will accommodate your needs, and allow you to sit on the floor with feet apart (turn the toes slightly inwards, and heel slightly outwards, for balance and comfort).

After you have established which of those positions described above will be most comfortable at this stage bend your upper body forward from the hips.

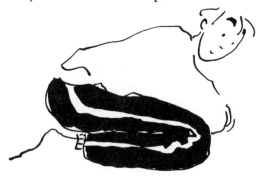

At this stage your buttocks will probably want to lift from the floor (or the cushion, or your feet); in time they will stay put. Slowly reach forward with arms outstretched so that your abdomen and chest come towards, and ideally touch and rest upon, your thighs, with your arms on the floor in front of you.

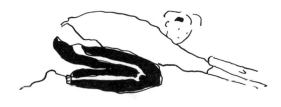

If this is not too difficult for you, then vary the hand position by placing them behind your back, palm to palm, as you do the slow forward bend.

Once you reach the limit of comfortable stretch, hold the position for between half a minute and a minute, while you do some slow deep breathing. Your head should be in line with your spine. There should be no pain at all, only a feeling of stretch. Come slowly out of this position, and go straight into the next exercises.

Advanced stretch 2

This is almost the reverse of the previous exercise. First, sit between your feet (or on them at first, or on a cushion, with feet apart and knees together, as in previous exercise). Slowly allow yourself to lean backwards, supporting yourself on your hands or elbows, until you reach the comfortable, tolerable limit of stretch available at this time.

If there is a limit to the distance you can stretch stop at that point and do the same for a minute or so. If there is any pain, especially in the back, then you are forcing the movement. It helps if you move the bones of the buttock area towards your knees, thus tilting your pelvis. The back and trunk should not be curved, but straight. Most of the movement and stretch should be localized in the hips and the front of the legs.

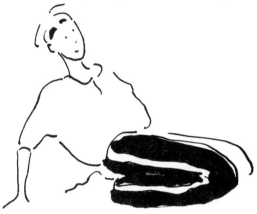

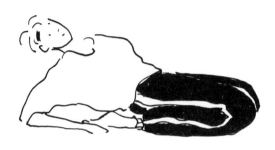

Use cushions behind you to support your various stages towards full stretch, if necessary. Do not force the pace, as there is nothing to be gained by not allowing the body its appropriate time to reach full stretch.

If you can go right back, to lie on the floor with your feet and lower legs still flat on the floor, and without undue strain , then just lie there and breathe deeply and relax.

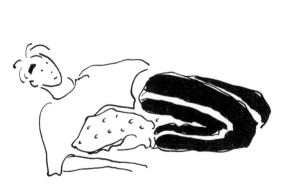

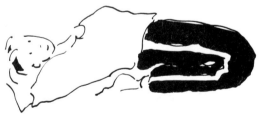

The adrenal type especially may never reach the full limits of any of these exercises. After a minute, or so, slowly come back to the upright position.

Advanced stretching 3

This is the final advanced stretching exercise, and completes the pattern of stretching as far as this programme is concerned.

Stand with your hands resting on your hips, and spread your legs apart about the distance of one good pace. Your right leg should be in front and your left leg behind. (This will be reversed after you have completed the first half of the exercise.)

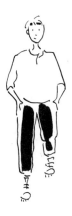

Turn the right foot to point straight in front of you. The left foot should be pointing outwards, but not at a right angle to the right foot, being turned slightly inwards, for balance. The centre of your left foot should be in a direct line behind your right heel. If this is so, then you should be nicely balanced.

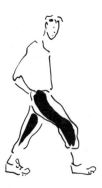

Adjust your weight so that it is centered over the left leg, and at the same time allow your upper body to lean to the right, from the hips, as far as it can comfortably go. Do not try to bend in the abdominal or chest area, just allow the body to lean as far as it can from the hips, keeping the upper body directly above the right leg as you do so. Keep the hips facing as they were when you started, as there will be a tendency to twist them towards the front. Turn your head to look upwards as you do this movement.

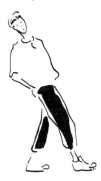

You should be aware of a strong, stretching feeling all down your left side to the waist, and down the inside of your right leg. Maintain this position for a minute or two, and then come slowly to an upright position, and change the whole thing around, so that the left leg is in front and you bend to the right, etc.

Check, as you do the stretch, that the distance between your legs is roughly equal to the length of one of your legs, and also that the front knee is pointing forward all the time. You should relax and breathe deeply during the performance of the exercise.

This is the minimum that is required to maintain mobility as we pass through the middle years of life. If you have found these exercises pleasurable and helpful, and (apart from the first few weeks) not too arduous, then join a yoga class, and develop this side of the programme.

Stretching summary

You have done the introductory bending-stretch, and the advanced stretching exercises, which completes this aspect of the exercise section. You will find that, by repetition, the performance of the set of stretching movements has a marvellously liberating effect on the way you feel. It also has a very important preparatory effect on the subsequent toning exercises.

It should not take you more than five minutes to do the set unless you add some of the basic stretching movements, which is a good idea if you have the time. Nor should it take you much less than five minutes, if you are doing them according to the instructions. The various types all benefit from these movements but the pituitary type enjoys them most and the adrenal type needs them most.

Remember that we must do these exercises at least five times a week. Even if you are not able to do the toning exercises (and these must be done at least every other day), you should try to complete the stretching and relaxing exercises. *Do not attempt to do the advanced stretching exercises unless you have been doing the basic stretching exercises for at least a month.*

Never do them in such a way as to cause pain. Discomfort is actually necessary, as a guide to the degree of stretch being achieved, but pain as such, is not, either during or after the exercises.

Never do the exercises immediately after a meal. Allow, if possible, one and a half hours after a meal before attempting them. A good time to do them, if you can so structure your life, is first thing in the morning. Many people however do them at the end of the day, and this does 'iron out' a few of the kinks and tensions built up in the hustle and bustle of modern life. After the stretching exercises we move as soon as possible to the toning exercise.

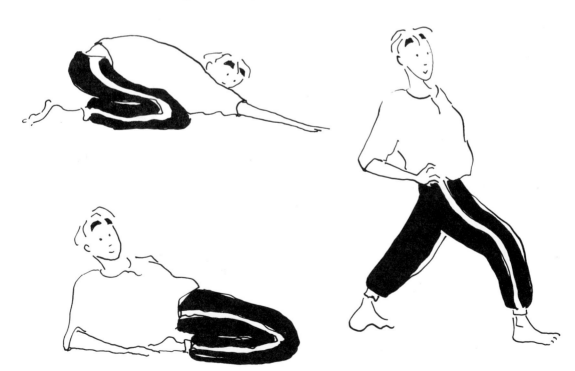

Toning exercise

The best advice anyone can be given, regarding toning or aerobic exercise, is that they walk!

Walking briskly is a wonderful toning exercise. Every muscle in the body is involved, and it makes the circulatory, and respiratory systems, speed up their activities marvellously.

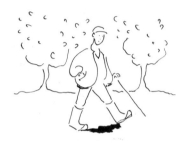

Apart from walking the other acceptable methods of toning are
- jogging,
- swimming,
- skipping,
- dancing,
- the use of indoor machines,
- or active sports.

From our point of view jogging has certain drawbacks for the unfit and the overweight, as it imposes a good deal of unnecessary strain on the weight bearing joints, such as the knees and hips.

Swimming requires special facilities and a lot of effort to gain the degree of toning that is required.

Indoor machines are fine, but take space and are expensive, as a rule. Also, the degree of effort involved is hard to monitor.

This leaves skipping and walking, as the safest activities, unless you play a game such as tennis or squash regularly (i.e. at least three times a week). The adrenal type enjoys competitive sport and may find this more attractive than walking.

On balance, therefore, I suggest walking, and perhaps skipping or dancing as the ideal methods of achieving, and then maintaining, your optimum fitness level. Dancing is also a good exercise and can replace walking and skipping from time to time.

Walking

Walking, if you walk you should do so at a brisk pace aiming to cover a distance of at least one mile, in about 15 minutes at the beginning. If you have been doing the initial ten minute walk a day, then you have probably been covering about three quarters of a mile a day. As you develop stamina, and as the weeks go by, you should aim to increase both your distance and your speed of walking.

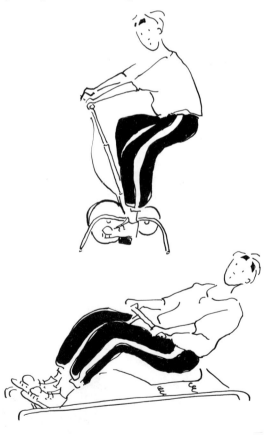

Monitor this by checking your pulse, and noting that you are indeed meeting your own physiological demands, as indicated by your fitness index.

At a rough guide you should, after a **month** of walking one mile a day (up to five times a week and not less than every other day), be aiming for a time of about 14 minutes. The **second month** should see you extending your distance by a half a mile to one-and-a-half miles, which you should cover in not more than 22 minutes, and probably not less than 21 minutes. At these *approximate* speeds you should find that your pulse rate will be reaching the levels required to maintain the toning process. If not you need to walk faster. The **third month** should see you aiming for two, to two-and-a-half miles, at each session, still averaging about 14 minutes per mile. Continue to increase your distance as you feel fitter, so that by the **fifth month** of the programme, you should reach your target of four miles at each session, and this total of four miles should be walked in the space of 56 minutes, thus maintaining your average of 14 minutes per mile for the whole distance.

Plan your route so that you are on level ground all the way and so that, if possible, you get some pleasant aspects to look at and clean air to breathe.

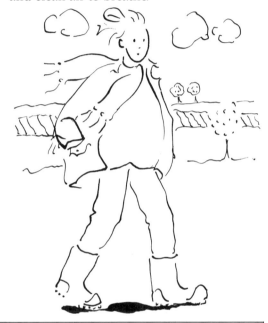

Pulse rate

Note: If you calculated your fitness index at the outset of the programme, as I asked you to in Chapter 4 then it is worth re-testing your waking pulse for three or more consecutive mornings. It may well have changed since the outset because, with the dietary and other changes, there could have been alterations in your metabolism which would reflect in the resting pulse rate. Recalculate in precisely, as indicated on page 50 and remember to re-check this important figure again in about three months time, as it could have altered further still, and this would give you new figures to remember when exercising. *Is the toning programme individualized?* Yes it is, in as much as it prescribes that you follow a particular pattern of exercise that is the same for all, but that you perform the exercise within guidelines that are set by your own physiology. The figures given for the amount of time that you should take to cover particular distances are averages, and I would expect that some people would achieve a one mile walk in an average of perhaps 12 minutes after a few months, whereas others may not achieve faster than 15 minutes per mile even after five months. As long as you are staying above the lower figure and below the upper figure of your fitness index, do not concern yourself more about speed of exercising.

Before you get too involved in the exercising go back to page 50 and recheck your sums as to what your two guiding figures are in relation to your pulse rate. You must get this right; remember, these are crucial numbers, one of which you must attempt to get beyond by your efforts, and one of which you must not exceed in your exercising. As you get fitter it will take more effort to get beyond the lower figure and be much harder to get anywhere near the upper figure. You will therefore be able to monitor your own constantly improving level of fitness.

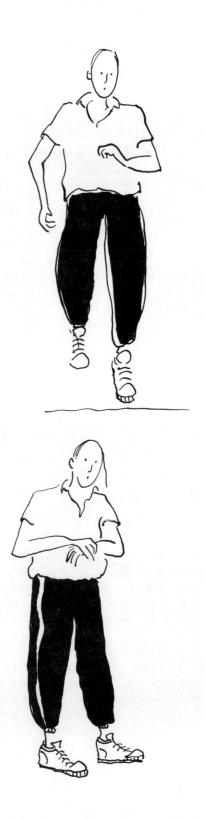

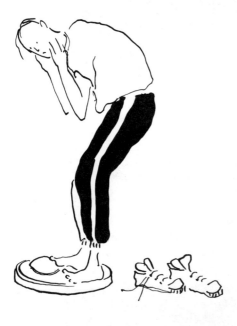

If you did nothing else on this whole programme, it is worth noting that the toning exercise alone would, over a year or so, reduce an overweight condition by upwards of fifteen pounds without any change in diet. But since our aim is health, as well as adjustment to your ideal weight, the diet is integral to the programme, and your achievements will be correspondingly greater.

Fitness and suppleness

There is no specific 'type' that will necessarily be able to achieve faster speeds within their safe limits of pulse rate although, generally speaking, the muscular tone and development of the adrenal type should give them great stamina. A 'mixed' type, who is unable to identify a dominant type in their make-up, is probably going to be the best athletic mix of stamina and speed.

It is not how fast you do the four mile walk that matters, but rather the fact that you achieve the distance regularly, while staying within the limits set by your fitness index.

You now have a programme of stretching exercise and toning exercise which you should build towards incorporating into your health and weight maintenance programme. Once you have been doing this for six months or so, you will be in a reasonable state of fitness and suppleness and you should continue to perform the programme at least three times weekly if you wish to maintain what you have worked so hard to achieve.

Once you have worked up to doing the full four mile work, you will be devoting an hour to the toning aspect of the programme every other day at least, and a further five minutes or so to your stretching exercises, although this should be more frequently performed than your toning exercise, and should always precede it.

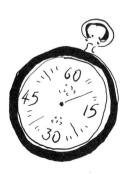

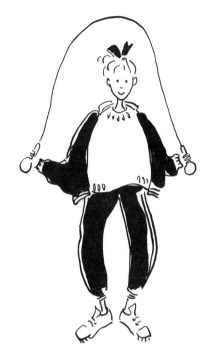

If walking is difficult, for one reason or another, then skipping will do in its place. This is something that you can do occasionally, instead of walking. The amount of continuous skipping that you must do to achieve the same degree of fitness as walking may surprise you. Fifteen minutes of continuous skipping will be roughly equal to a mile walk. So, on days that you cannot go for a walk, you could achieve your target by skipping for two sessions of ten minutes or so. Do not forget to monitor your pulse rate, as this is a more concentrated form of exercise.

When you first introduce skipping, start with only a few minutes and gradually increase, so that after a month you can skip non-stop for ten minutes. After two months you should be able to do 15 minutes, non-stop, within your fitness index limits. Do not base your toning programme on skipping, but use it as a substitute for those times when you cannot fit a walk into your schedule.

Relaxation

You should have been following the rhythmic breathing exercise as set out on page 43, for at least a month before introducing the following exercise in guided imagery or visualization into your programme. By now you are aware of your physical and emotional type more clearly than you were at the outset, especially if you have been able to identify a dominant characteristic which places you in one group or another. If you have not, you will have identified aspects of yourself in all of the types, and this is an insight in itself.

Visualization

After doing the rhythmic breathing exercise I want you to lie very still and to feel a sense of contentment, of wholeness and of peace. This is the result of your own efforts towards meeting your unique biochemical and metabolic needs. You are also beginning to meet exercise requirements which are to be performed at a rate unique to your needs. Your emotional needs are no less unique than these others. For perhaps the first time in many years you are beginning to give to yourself those factors which your individuality requires, to function at its best level. This is a momentous turning point in your life. You are beginning to control your own destiny in terms of health and well-being, and from this can flow untold benefits in terms of happiness and a successful life, in the best sense of that word.

Is it selfish, this concentration on self? This is often asked, and I categorically reject the idea. If you are to be of use to others in life, then you must be able to function adequately. If that takes a certain amount of time devoted to meeting your inborn requirements, it is still anything but selfish. Of course it could become so if that was all you ever thought about, and if you saw your goal of optimum health and

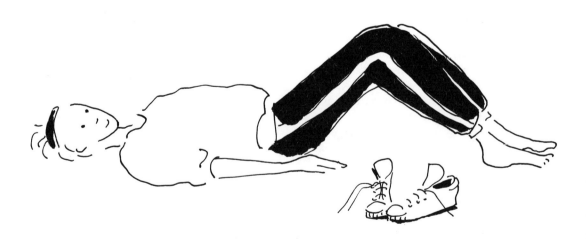

weight as the end of the story. I believe that well people are usually happy people. Happy people are good for the world and good for other people, and this is our ultimate hope and goal. Once you are healthy and at peace with yourself, you can forget about your particular needs for most of each day (not all of it, though, as maintenance must continue). When that stage is reached you can devote your health, energy and happiness to anything that you wish, knowing that your body and mind are harmoniously in tune, and your abilities will be greater in any direction than they ever were before you achieved this invaluable state.

Visualization requires that you exercise your powers of imagination. To do this you first spend a few minutes doing the deep rhythmic breathing exercise as outlined on page 43. Having reached a point of contented stillness of mind, introduce into your mind a picture of a place in which you could feel happy and safe.

This can be a room, a country or garden scene, or any place in which you could see yourself, and which will help to instill a sense of security and safety. By exercising your imaginative powers you should be able to visualize this place in such a way as to allow you to step into or out of it at will. The picture should not be static.

It should contain as many elements of your senses as you can manage. Thus, in a country garden you should be able to smell flowers, feel the breeze, hear the birds and sense the warmth of the sun, as well as seeing the variety of trees and flowers that will complete the image. This can be varied from time to time with different scenes but many people enjoy the regular return to a real or imaginary place, which some have called their 'corner of heaven'. It has also been described as a 'safe haven', to which we can retreat in times of stress, so that the mind has respite from the turmoil of its problems. The object, at this stage, is for you to find such a place, and to exercise your powers of imagination regularly by spending a period of about two minutes there before going on to the guided visualization exercise proper.

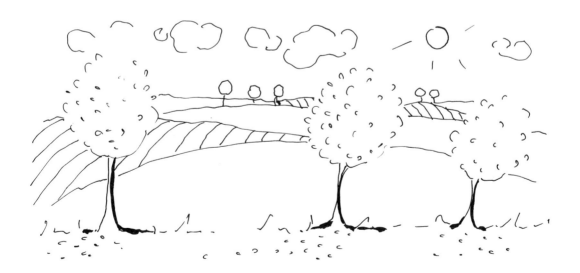

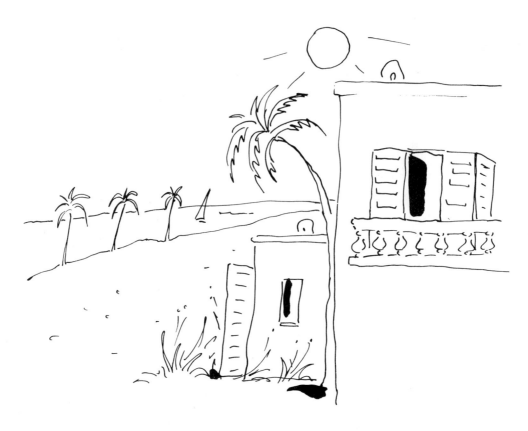

You may well find that stray thoughts enter your mind as you attempt this initial trip into conscious day-dreaming. This is to be expected, and is part of the reason for your doing the exercise. You are learning to guide your mind to a particular thought pattern and, in doing so, your usual random thought patterns will intrude. All you need to do when you become conscious of this is to gently replace the thought that has intruded with the image that you have decided upon as your 'safe haven'.

Remember also that many people have less well-developed imaginative powers than others. The actual seeing of the imagined scene as though it were a film on a screen may not be possible to some, at first. It may be easier to imagine the scene verbally, or as a series of ideas. It doesn't matter at all.

What is important is that you begin to guide your mind to a particular place, and that this is seen as vividly as possible in whatever way your unique imaginative faculty can achieve. As with any new experience it takes time to become familiar with the process.

In time you may well find that you can swiftly establish a clear visual image of the place and can then add the other dimensions of sound, feelings, smell, etc. Take your time and enjoy the trip. Its limitations depend only upon your willingness to explore the inner space of your mind's imaginative facility.

After a few minutes of this exercise you should proceed to the guided imagery exercise.

Guided imagery or visualization

This simply means that you are leading your mind to visualize certain predetermined images which are supportive of your health or other goals in life.

Visualize or imagine a state of health exactly as you wish it to be. This may mean seeing yourself as slimmer, more active, healthier and energetic. See the desired state as being possible, and know for certain that it is achievable by the methods you have already adopted, and which you are faithfully pursuing. See the goals as attainable by these means, and know that this is not a far-fetched dream but a practical reality which is the natural consequence of what you are doing.

As you visualize yourself in an active, healthy, vital manner, make certain positive statements such as: 'I am slim and supple and healthy', or 'I feel well, energetic and happy' or 'My body is strong, and full of energy'. The importance of such affirmations cannot be over-emphasized (choose any that suit your particular needs at the time). They should always be phrased as positive statements, so that you would say, 'I feel energetic', rather than, 'I no longer feel tired', which contains negative aspects.

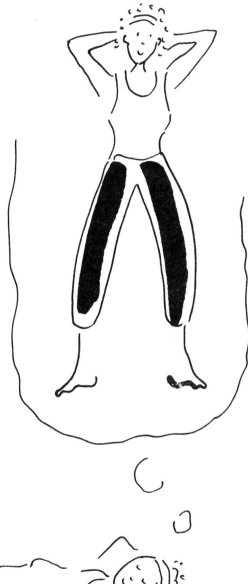
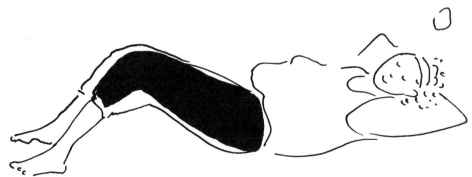

The phrase you choose should have a comfortable feel to you as you verbalize it. So you are seeing, in your mind's eye, the image of yourself as you believe you can be and you are affirming verbally, in appropriate ways, the reality of this belief. You also are seeing that what you are doing in the way of diet and exercise is having its effects upon your health, weight, etc. You can visualize the exercises making your body supple and fit; the diet and supplements providing your body with its precise nutrient needs, and resulting in a healthier, more appropriate structure. The whole programme is seen as giving a new direction and purpose to your life.

The value and success of this exercise is limited only by your powers of imagery, and by your application of these. There is no condition of health that cannot be improved by these methods, and no pattern of ill health that cannot be thus assisted towards recovery. The pattern remains the same, only the images and affirmations need to alter with varying needs.

Now it is most important that you have realistic images in order to achieve success. If you were to imagine that you were flying like a bird, then no amount of imagery, or affirmation, would ever help in the accomplishment of this goal. You must have a goal which is realistically attainable, and which you are doing someting positive to achieve.

Once you have established clearly what your realistic goals of health and weight are, then they are certainly achievable by a combination of positive action (the programme) and your mind's co-operative effort, as evidenced by the visualization exercise. 'I am well, energetic and happy'. These are goals we can justifiably aim for, and which our efforts will ensure.

The relative degree of slimness is going to flow from these efforts, but will, to some extent, be determined by your metabolic type. So, if you have established that you are an adrenal type, and that your normal, healthy weight is above the average for your height, then programme your visualization accordingly. Be happy with the way nature

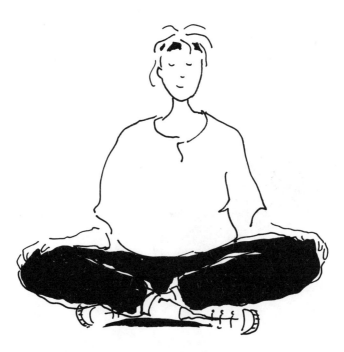

made you, and aim for your ideal figure, and optimum health level. It is probably best therefore if, in your imagery, and your accompanying verbal statements, you have an image of health, and vitality, rather than of a very slim you, which your metabolic type may preclude. Have realistic and achievable goals, and use the power of the mind to support your efforts towards this end.

This exercise should be done daily. Altogether it requires about five to seven minutes of your time:
- the breathing exercise to relax you;
- the 'safe haven' image, and then
- the guided visualization of your aims and desires.

A good time to do the exercise is before a meal. It will relax you and aid your digestion, as well as being part of a pattern of activity that will help to establish it as a regular routine. Regularity is the key to its success, as is the case with the toning and stretching exercises. By finding an appropriate time of day, and sticking to it, you will soon automatically fit it into your life pattern. Do not do the exercise immediately after a meal.

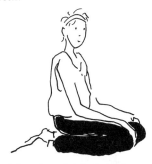

The position in which it is done is unimportant as long as you are comfortable, without distraction or muscular strain. Lying on the floor or a bed is fine, so long as you stay awake. Sitting on the floor, kneeling or squatting are also acceptable. Be warm, unrushed, and undisturbed during the exercise.

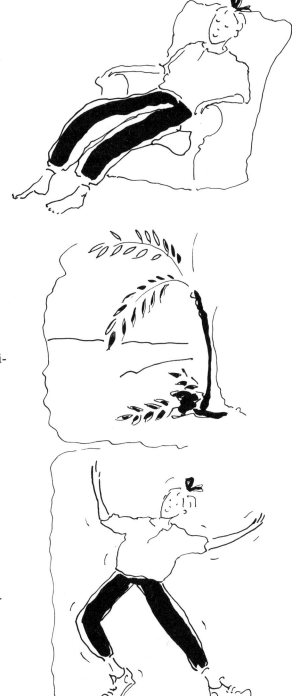

Timing

You now have the three elements of your exercise programme.

Stretching, (daily if possible, and always preceding the toning exercise).

Toning exercise (three times a week, minimum).

Relaxation/guided imagery exercise (daily). This latter is done at a separate time from the others.

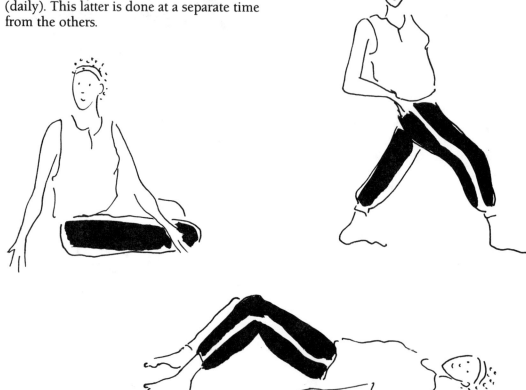

At first you need ten minutes for the stretching exercise and 15 for the toning exercise, with five to seven for the relaxation/guided imagery. As you progress the only one that will require more time is the toning exercise, as your distance increases. So the time you have to give up to the programmes needs involve at least half an hour, at first, on the days that you are doing the toning exercise, and 15 minutes on the days that you are not. As time goes by this will mean that on three or four days a week you need to devote an hour and a quarter to the programmes exercise requirement, and 15 minutes daily on the days on which toning (aerobic walking) is not in the schedule.

Regularity and persistance will soon make these elements of the programme so important a part of your life that you would not dream of missing them.

Endocrine dysfunctions

This chapter is concerned with the over-or under-function of particular endocrine glands, and this can happen no matter which 'type' you fit into. Thus you may find that you are showing evidence of an underactive thyroid gland, whilst having managed to categorize yourself as an adrenal type. *Any type can have any particular manifestation of dysfunction,* which gives us quite a few permutations to consider.

Having ascertained whether you are an adrenal, pituitary, thyroid or mixed type, you will be aware of the pattern of eating, and the general supplements, indicated for your particular biochemical needs. This will be modified by what you discover in this chapter, if the indications are that one or other of the endocrine glands, is over-or under-functioning. It is necessary to evolve your final pattern of eating and supplementation in this manner, as we must superimpose the alterations called for by possible dysfunction, onto the pattern broadly indicated by your metabolic type.

You will recall the two tests that you were asked to complete in Chapter 4. I would like you to do them again, now that you have spent some time on the basic diet and exercise programme. There may have been a change since the beginning of your involvement in the programme, showing that your biological needs have been met at least in part resulting in positive physiological alterations.

Do the underarm temperature test again (page 47) and the lying down, and standing up, blood-pressure test as well (if you can, find a practitioner to do this for you) as described on page 48.

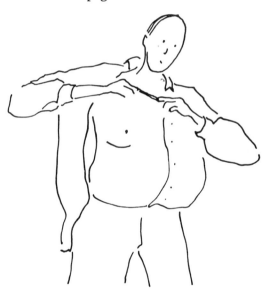

Use the results of these tests to confirm the findings which you will come to after completing the following questionnaires. Before embarking on the changes suggested as a result of such findings, check the questionnaires carefully to be sure that you have answered accurately. Repeat the tests every three months to see if the endocrine dysfunction has improved or is now no longer a factor in your life.

Once you can see that the questionnaires and tests indicate a balanced endocrine system, simply revert to the programme as indicated for your type. There is sometimes confusion over whether your type has anything to do with the sort of dysfunction we are trying to assess in this chapter. In fact it does but, as far as our concern goes, all that you need to do is to alter your programme slightly depending upon what shows up in the questionnaires that follow.

Your type to some extent determines the way you live your life, and that, to a large extent, will influence the functioning of your endocrine glands. This is especially true of the adrenal glands, which can be devastated by a combination of stress, high sugar intake and the use of common stimulants (tea, coffee, chocolate, alcohol, cigarettes, drugs, etc).

These glands are the source of vital hormonal substances which control our well-being, and which we must protect and conserve if we are to reach a reasonable level of health.

It is also important to note that overfunction of an organ or gland often precedes its collapse into underfunctioning. If, therefore, you find one or other of the questionnaires leads to the conclusion that a gland is overfunctioning, this is just as important to our purpose as finding the opposite. You will realize from the questions themselves just what sort of influences these two glands can have.

There are, of course, many factors which can disturb the function of the body, other than the dysfunction of these two glands. They are, however, pertinent to our quest, and are open to assistance by dietary methods, at least in the early stages of dysfunction. We will highlight other aspects of the health picture in subsequent questionnaires, after you have sorted out these two major areas, the thyroid and the adrenal glands.

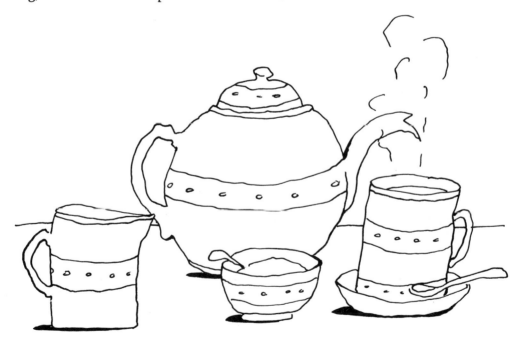

Thyroid function

Confirm by means of the following questions and answers whether you have an underactive thyroid (average of three days early morning underarm temperature test below 97.8°F/36.5°C) or an overactive thyroid (above 98.2°F/36.8°C).

Overactive thyroid questionnaire

Answer the following *yes* if the description applies to you once a week or more; *sometimes* if twice a month or more, but less than weekly, and *seldom* if once a month or less. Score two for 'yes', one for 'sometimes', none for 'seldom'.

1. Have you a very big appetite?
2. Are you disturbed by heat, and/or do you enjoy a cool or chilly atmosphere?
3. Do you blush easily?
4. Do you have night sweats?
5. Are you aware of an inner trembling?
6. Does your heart race, and beat strongly even when you are at rest?
7. Are you irritable and restless?
8. Do your eyelids or face twitch?
9. Are you highly emotional, or nervous?
10. Is your skin frequently moist?
11. Do you suffer from insomnia?
12. Is it normally hard for you to gain weight?

If your underarm test indicates an overactive thyroid, and your score in the above test is six or more, then your thyroid is probably overactive. This can sometimes cause overweight problems as well as underweight, since there is frequently an increase in appetite which can lead to overeating and thus obesity. In this condition, a person is often referred to as being a 'fast metabolizer'. The additional supplements indicated are as follows:

Vitamin A
B Complex
Calcium orotate
Potassium orotate
Thymus gland
Kelp

(For quantities see page 115.)

If the underarm test is not confirmed by the questionnaire or if the questionnaire is not confirmed by the underarm test, ignore them in so far as the additional supplements are concerned. There can be other reasons for such symptoms, unrelated to thyroid function, and these should be taken care of by the general pattern described in previous chapters, together with the suggestions resulting from your individual assessment of your health status.

Underactive thyroid questionnaire

1. Does your weight increase easily?
2. Has your appetite been depressed?
3. Do you tire easily?
4. Do you get ringing in the ears?
5. Do you feel sleepy during the day?
6. Is your skin thick, dry or scaly?
7. Are you sensitive to the cold?
8. Do you suffer from constipation?
9. Is your hair coarse and falling, or are the outer third of your eyebrows thin?
10. Do you need to urinate frequently?
11. Is your pulse slow (below 65 per minute)?
12. Do you feel sluggish and lacking in drive?

Again, answer with a 'yes', 'sometimes', or 'seldom', and score two, one or none accordingly. If the total for this questionnaire is six points or more, and your underarm temperature average for three consecutive days was below 97.8°F (36.5°C), then you probably have an underactive thyroid, and your additional supplement needs are, as follows:

Kelp (for iodine)
Copper orotate
Zinc orotate
Tyrosine
Vitamin B complex
Dolomite tablets (calcium/magnesium)
Vitamin F (Evening Primrose Oil)
Thyroid gland extract

(For quantities see pages 115.)

(If the tests do not confirm each other then ignore these additional supplements).

Repeat the questionnaires and tests after three months, and discontinue the supplements if the tests do not still indicate either an over-or underactive thyroid. If this is the case simply continue with the programme as indicated by your metabolic type or, if this is not clearly indentifiable, then continue on the basic diet together with particular nutrients, as may be indicated in the following chapter.

Your exercise and visualization pattern continues unchanged as you make these nutritional adjustments.

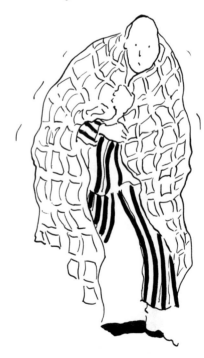

Adrenal function

The next set of questionnaires examines the possibility of your adrenal glands being over-or underactive, and the findings of the questionnaire should be confirmed by the standing/lying blood-pressure tests, as far as an underactive adrenal function is concerned. This means that if you produce a result in the questionnaire that indicates poor adrenal function, then your systolic blood-pressure should show a failure to rise by at least five points from lying down blood-pressure to that registered when standing up.

There is no simple test for an overactive adrenal function and we must rely on the questionnaire. In the case of overactive adrenals, however, we would only suggest additional supplementation if the questionnaire score is eight, or higher. The scoring for this questionnaire is the same as for those previously.

Underactive adrenal function questionnaire

1. Do you lack energy, and feel generally fatigued, or wake with headaches?
2. Do you have any allergies?
3. Do you have a noticeable lack of saliva?
4. Is your circulation poor: i.e., cold hands and feet?
5. Do sugary, starchy foods cause you to have indigestion?
6. Do you like salty foods?
7. Do beans, cabbage or Brussels sprouts give you indigestion?
8. If you rise quickly from a chair do you feel dizzy or faint?
9. Do your ankles swell at night, or have you any fluid retention?
10. Do you find yourself yawning, sighing and constantly requiring fresh air?
11. Do you find you are frequently ill with colds and minor infections?
12. Are your nails ridged?

If you score six or more in the above questionnaire and your blood-pressure test indicates an underactive adrenal function as described on page 48, then you probably have a need to assess your overall stress levels. It is clear from numerous studies that stress is one of the key reasons for the development of what has come to be called 'adrenal exhaustion'. There is a great deal that you can do about this and, by following the programme thus far, the dietary pattern, the nutrient supplements, the exercise patterns and the relaxation/visualization programme, you will already be achieving a great deal. In addition, you should take the following supplements for the next three months, before reassessing yourself as to your adrenal function:
Calcium pantothenate (500 mg)
'Strong' vitamin B complex tablet
Vitamin C
2 × 150 mg adrenal glandular extract daily
(For quantities refer to page 115.)

Stress reduction

In addition, the following stress-reducing factors may be worth looking at and adopting if called for with an underactive adrenal function.

- Avoid working more than ten hours daily and ensure that you have at least 1 day a week free of routine work. If at all possible, an annual holiday 'away from it all' should be arranged.

- During each day, have at least two relaxation or meditation periods. Time should be set aside morning and evening, or just prior to a meal.

- Perform active physical exercise for at least ten minutes daily, or for 20-minute periods four times each week.

- Balance the diet and eliminate stress-inducing foods and drinks.

- Try to move, talk and behave in a relaxed manner.

- Seek advice about any sexual or emotional problems that are nagging away at the back of your mind, or which are causing conscious anxiety.

- If there are actual stress-inducing factors at work or home, which can be altered, then make concrete steps towards these changes.

- Cultivate a creative rather than a competitive hobby, e.g. painting, DIY, gardening, etc.

- Try to live in the present, avoiding undue reflection on past events or anticipating possible future ones.

- Concentrate on whatever the current task is, always finishing one thing before starting another.

- Avoid making deadlines or 'impossible' promises that could lead to stress. Take on only what you can happily cope with.

- Learn to express feelings openly in a non-belligerent way and, in turn, learn to listen carefully to other people.

- Accept personal responsibility for your life and health—don't look outside yourself for causes or cures, apart from the objective guidance and practical advice available from a health professional.

- Greet, smile at and respond towards people in the same way that you would like to be treated.

- Introduce negative ionization into the home or work place and ensure adequate exposure to full-spectrum light.

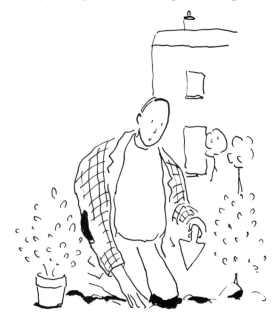

Overactive adrenal function questionnaire

1. Do you suffer from daytime headaches?
2. Do you have high blood-pressure (over 145 systolic and over 90 diastolic)?
3. Do you suffer from an 'acid' stomach (heartburn, gastritis, etc.)?
4. Do you suffer from spastic constipation?
5. Do you have a high sex-drive?
6. Do you have apparently unlimited energy?
7. Are you aggressive, with very strong feelings?
8. Do you have difficulty getting to sleep?
9. Have you noticed an increased growth of hair?
10. Do you have a rapid heart beat (above 80)?
11. Do you suffer from backaches, other than caused by injury?
12. Do you suffer from dizziness, other than when getting up from a sitting position?

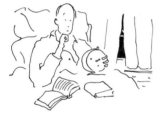

The scoring for this questionnaire is the same as for those previously. Having a score of eight or more on this questionnaire indicates a probability of an overactive adrenal function, which in time could result in adrenal exhaustion, and consequent underfunction. Take the following supplements for the next three months:

Kelp
Manganese orotate
B complex
2 × 150 mg adrenal extract
Vitamin C
Calcium pantothenate

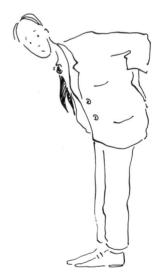

Take these in addition to any that you are already taking, or which might be indicated in the following chapter, up to the limits on page 115.

Use of supplements

The following chapter is concerned with the use of nutritional supplements.

You are already doing a great deal about correcting the underlying causes of any dysfunction, by means of the diet, exercise and visualization programmes that you are following.

The additional aid to be derived from the supplements suggested will help in the normalization of the condition, and in your gaining a sense of well-being and health. All of the foregoing conditions can be related to overweight, or they may exist in a body which is maintaining its weight balance adequately.

The primary aim, in correcting mild endocrine dysfunction, is to help to achieve a better overall level of health from which will flow the normalization of any weight problem which may be accompanying it. Our primary aim is health. This is the key to success in the weight adjustment that may be desirable in your particular case.

You have now identified your metabolic type, and are meeting the specific needs indicated by that type. You are also following an exercise pattern which, by monitoring your pulse rate, is specifically tuned to your current needs. You are also following a pattern of relaxation and visualization, which is also personal in that you are setting your own goals and are visualizing these.

Now you may have identified particular idiosyncracies, which require correction, in your endocrine system. There may, of course, be no problems at all, as indicated by the tests or the questionnaires. If this is the case then ignore the additional advice in this chapter and go on the following one, which will identify particular nutrient needs (if any) based on your accurate answering of a series of specific health questions.

If you have identified any of the dysfunctions in this chapter as being related to you then may I repeat the instruction that you should follow the nutrient supplement suggestion for at least three months, as well as the programme identified in previous chapters. Reassess the endocrine (thyroid or adrenal) function in three months, and either continue or stop, as indicated. But do continue with the programme as a whole, as well as any nutrients indicated in the next chapter.

We will now pass on to the last of our assessments, which you should read carefully as we are looking for ways of identifying aspects of your unique biochemical requirements, over and above those indicated by your particular type. If at any time there is a duplication of nutrient indication, then follow instructions on page 115, regarding what dosages are applicable when there are multiple indications for particular nutrients.

Note:
The advice given in the next chapter should not preclude your taking expert professional advice. The advice is meant to complement a complete health enhancement programme and should not be taken out of context, or in isolation from that programme.

Further nutritional needs

Whilst important to your overall health programme, the following advice contained in this chapter is not essential unless the symptoms and signs mentioned in the questions are marked and obvious. If the questions do not seem to apply to you ignore them and continue to the next section.

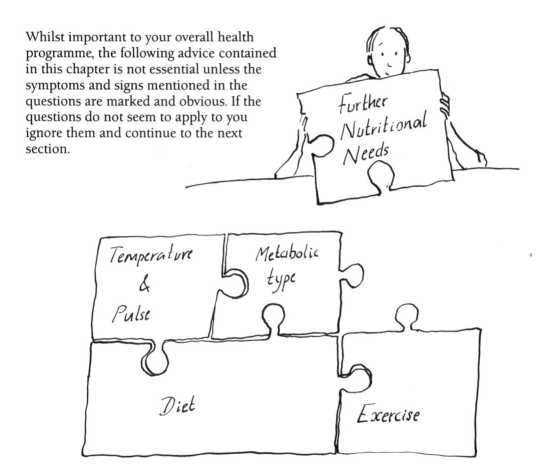

In this chapter we are going, by means of questionnaires, to identify those aspects of your biochemical make-up that are currently not being met by your diet. It will give us information which, combined with the indications derived from the tests (morning underarm temperature test; lying and standing blood-pressure test) and questionnaires that you have done in the previous chapter, will allow the prescribing of nutrient supplements which will assist your body in its normalization process. This is the final piece in our 'jig-saw puzzle' of individualizing your dietary and nutrient pattern, as part of the overall programme that will lead to optimum health and weight.

You should by now have done the following:

- Abandoned the 'tasty toxins'.

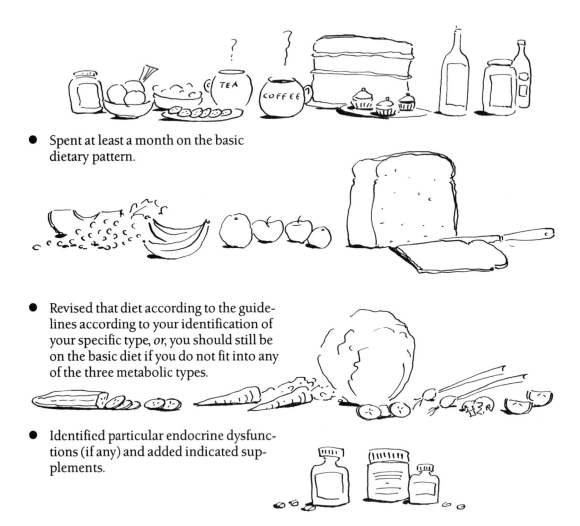

- Spent at least a month on the basic dietary pattern.

- Revised that diet according to the guidelines according to your identification of your specific type, *or*, you should still be on the basic diet if you do not fit into any of the three metabolic types.

- Identified particular endocrine dysfunctions (if any) and added indicated supplements.

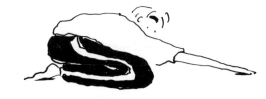

- Spent a month or so on the introductory stretching exercises, basic toning exercise, and rhythmic breathing exercise, and then have modified all of those to the advanced levels. You should be monitoring your toning exercise by reference to your fitness index. This pattern should by now also include the use of the guided imagery exercise.

Now you are going to identify those aspects of your individual biochemical requirements which need attention, via the use of either dietary changes or the short term (i.e. six months or so) use of supplements.

After six months or so on the full programme, starting from the implementation of the suggestions made in this chapter, you should reassess everything that has determined your programme, although it will only be three months for your first endocrine reassessment. You must re-do the questionnaires, the tests, the fitness index, etc., and see what has changed. The subsequent six months should then be spent on the revised programme which you will determine from the new results and answers. You should find that your fitness index has changed, as your resting pulse rate will be different from when you started. You should also notice differences in the answers you give to the questions in this chapter, and very likely there will be changes in the results of the underarm temperature test, and the blood-pressure test, too. This will be dramatic evidence of the power of your body to respond positively to a health improvement programme whic takes account of what it really needs.

You will notice that, for some of the questions in this section, I have given an explanation of what the answer means, and why a particular nutrient is indicated. In some I have not done so because the explanations are too complex, and a number of answers give an indication of a trend, rather than a specific and directly applicable clue.

Answer the questions honestly and follow the advice as given. These indicators are vital to your health programme. You can achieve wonders with the dietary pattern alone and, as I have said, the exercise programme of toning and stretching would revolutionize your life on its own. Together

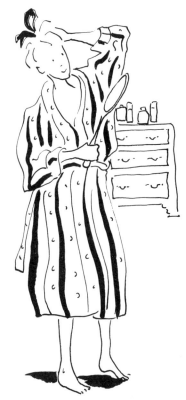

they are a marvellous team, and they are reinforced by the use of the nutrients for which your body shows specific need.

There is no quicker way of revitalizing the body than by the provision of those nutrients which it needs and which are deficient in the diet. Do not forget that some needs may have been under-fulfilled for a considerable time—perhaps even since birth. It takes some months of using supplements, as directed, before reasonable levels of these nutrients are absorbed into the system, and the metabolism begins to respond by better function. Do not expect immediate results. You will find that by looking back over a six month period, however, and comparing the answers as given at the outset with your new results, you will prove the value of what you have been doing. You should feel fitter, have more energy, be more alert and vital, and hopefully be slimmer, than at the outset.

Nutritional questionnaire

As you answer these questions note which supplements are suggested in response to your answers. You will see that in most cases no quantities are given. After answering all thirty questions, and the final health indicator question, you should then refer to the list of supplements at the end of the questionnaire. Here you will find the quantities that should be *added* to your overall programme. These are calculated upon the number of times you have answered questions in such a way as to suggest the particular supplement as necessary.

Thus you may for example answer yes to questions 21 and 22. Both of these indicate that you should take thiamin (as well as other nutrients). Having two indications for thiamin you should take a dosage of 50mg daily, as a supplement. If there had been only one 'yes' response then your dosage should be 25 mg daily.

You will see from the supplement recommendation list that this is not an ever-expanding ratio. You will find, for example, that many of the answers indicate a need for a 'strong' vitamin B complex tablet (see page 118 for details of stockists, etc.)

You require three affirmatives before you are requested to take two of these tablets and, no matter how many more than that are indicated by your score, you will not be required to take more than two.

It may sound complicated, but in fact only requires that you answer your questions and keep 'score'. After that, consult the supplement quantity list and all will become clear to you. If any of the supplements indicated in this section are already being taken, because of indications regarding your endocrine pattern or metabolic type, they are taken into account when fixing your daily intake levels.

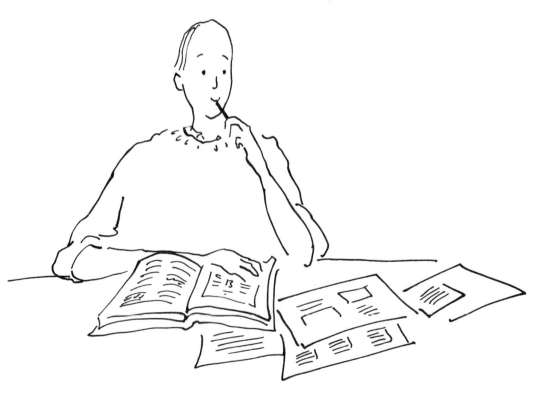

Read the questions carefully and answer frankly:

1. **Do you believe your body weight to be 20lb (9 kilos) or more above your ideal weight for height ratio?**

If so supplement your dietary programme with Vitamin C.

2. **Are you a smoker, or are you exposed to a smoky atmosphere at work or at home?**

If the answer is yes then take 500mg daily of methionine (amino acid) and also vitamin C and vitamin A (in the form of beta-carotene). Try to stop smoking.

3. **Do you live, or work, in an environment that is known to be polluted by industrial or automobile fumes?**

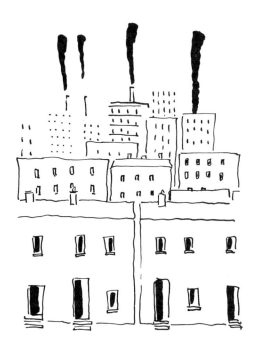

If the answer is yes then take additional vitamin C, beta-carotene (vitamin A), vitamin E, selenium, and 1g of glutathione (an amino acid complex). These are all antioxidants, which will protect you from the damage that can result from exposure to pollutants.

4. **Do you react very rapidly to alcohol, i.e., become red in the face and feel happy or 'woozy', more quickly than is usual?**

If so then you are probably metabolizing the alcohol poorly, and your liver is having trouble detoxifying and eliminating the products of the metabolism. You should refrain from all alcohol for the next six months, and add the following to your supplement list: zinc orotate (B_{13} zinc), strong B complex (see note at end of chapter regarding the way to choose supplements).

5. **Are you very sensitive to changes of temperatures?**

If so, then take kelp (for iodine), zinc orotate (B_{13} zinc) and tyrosine (an amino acid).

6. **Do you crave sweet food?**

If so then you need a strong B complex supplement and zinc orotate (B_{13} zinc).

7. **Does your hair lack in quality, or do you have dandruff?**

If so then add the following to your programme: strong B complex and selenium. Make sure that you are eating adequate protein (if you are of northern European stock then you may need as much as 100g (4 oz) of protein daily—either of animal or vegetable origin, depending upon your metabolic type; if you are of Oriental or Middle Eastern origin, then you may be adequately nourished on as little as 50g (2 oz) of protein daily).

8. Have you a history of mild allergies, such as hayfever?

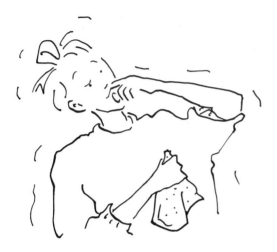

If so then add to your programme: vitamin B_6; manganese orotate (B_{13} manganese), and calcium pantothenate (vitamin B_5).

9. Are you aware of small broken veins beneath the skin, or redness of the whites of the eyes?
If so add bioflavonoids and vitamin C; strong B complex and vitamin E.

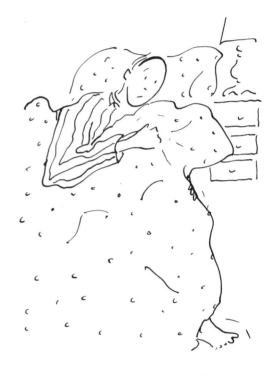

10. Are your lips frequently chapped, or do you often have cracks at the corner of your mouth?
Take strong vitamin B complex, if so.

11. Is the skin along the backs of your arms rough, and flaky in texture?
If so take emulsified (or miscible) vitamin A.

12. Are you prone to cramps at night, or do your legs feel uncomfortable and difficult to find a position of ease?
If so take strong B complex, vitamin E and zinc orotate (B_{13} zinc). Also calcium orotate (B_{13} calcium) and magnesium orotate (B_{13} magnesium).

13. Is your tongue bright red, and very smooth?
Add vitamin B_2 and vitamin B_3 as well as a strong B complex tablet.

14. Has your sense of taste and/or smell become noticeably less acute?
If so then you are probably zinc deficient, and a supplement is indicated. This is obtained by taking zinc orotate (B_{13} zinc). In addition add vitamin A to your programme.

15. Do you see poorly at night?
If so make sure that you get adequate yellow and orange coloured fruits and vegetables, and take emulsified (miscible) vitamin A daily.

16. Do you have recurrent head noises of a buzzing or ringing type?

This can be because of the taking of aspirin; if not then add magnesium orotate (B_{13} magnesium) and manganese orotate (B_{13} manganese).

17. Is your memory less than adequate, and have you noticed this yourself?

If so then add 1000 milligrams of lecithin; strong B complex and calcium and manganese (in the form of B_{13} calcium and B_{13} manganese).

18. Do you have greasy flakes of skin on the forehead, or around the nose or mouth?

If so take vitamin B_6.

19. Do your gums bleed easily when being brushed?

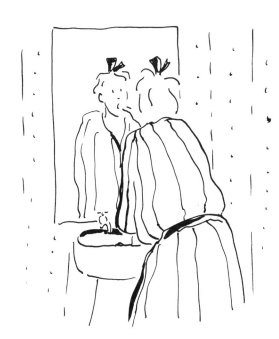

If the answer is yes, then add vitamin C, bioflavonoids and folic acid.

20. Is your mouth very sensitive to hot drinks?

If so add strong B complex.

21. Do your tongue or lips feel a burning sensation?

If so then add vitamin B_1 (thiamin) to your programme as well as strong B complex.

22. Do you feel sensations of tingling, or burning, in your hands or feet?

If so this may indicate a form of nerve irritation (sometimes produced by excessive tea drinking) which requires the addition to your programme of Vitamin B_1 (thiamin) and B_2 (riboflavin) as well as another of the B vitamins called inositol, at a dosage of between 500 and 1000 milligrams. All these should be taken with a strong B complex tablet.

23. Look at your nails and note whether they show ridges, or white flecks, or spots.

If so then you require to supplement with iron and calcium and zinc. Ensure that you add vitamin C to your programme at each main meal (2g daily), to improve the intake of iron from your food. Also ensure that if you drink tea (and you shouldn't be having much, if any) then it is not a meal times, as this upsets iron absorption. Also add zinc orotate (B_{13} zinc) to your programme as well as calcium orotate (B_{13} calcium). If, after three months, the nails are not noticably improved, in terms of the ridging, then start a supplementation of iron (as iron orotate— B_{13} iron). Take the iron and zinc at separate times as they compete for absorption.

24. **Can you remember your dreams upon waking?**
If not then there is a strong possibility that you are low in your levels of vitamin B_6. This should be supplemented as well as strong B complex.

25. **Is your skin very oily, with enlarged pores?**
If so then vitamins B_2 (riboflavin) and B_6 (pyridoxine) are indicated, as well as strong B complex.

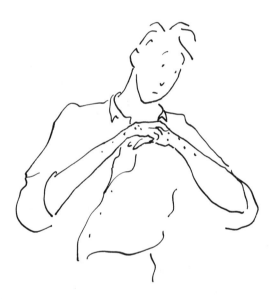

26. **Do you have 'age spots' such as brown, or yellowish, fatty growths on the skin?**
Chromium and vitamin C are both indicated. Take chromium orotate (B_{13} chromium) as well as vitamin C. If any difficulty is experienced obtaining a chromium supplement then take a minimum of 9 brewer's yeast tablets daily, with food, as a source of this most important mineral.

27. **Do you suffer from insomnia?**
If you have difficulty in going to sleep, and in staying asleep, then you are probably in need of vitamin B_6, magnesium and the amino acid tryptophan. These have been combined as a compound called Sonnamin (made by the Cantassium Co.; see note regarding suppliers of nutrient supplements on page 118). If unavailable take 15mg vitamin B_6, 500 mg magnesium orotate, and 750 mg tryptophan, half an hour before retiring.

28. **Do you actually burn when in the sun, rather than tanning?**
If so then take a supplement of the B-complex element called PABA (para-aminobenzoic acid) of 1000mg daily; also vitamin B_6 and vitamin B_3 (niacin or niacinamide) as well as beta-carotene daily (pro-vitamin A).

29. **Do you get shaky if you miss a meal?**
It may indicate a tendency to what is termed hypoglycaemia, and this should be corrected by the programme that you are now on. Add manganese orotate (B_{13} manganese) and three brewer's yeast tablets with each main meal (9 daily) as a source of B vitamins and chromium (which is a part of the Glucose Tolerance Factor).

30. **Do you suffer from indigestion after eating a protein meal?**
If so this can indicate a tendency for the pancreas to be underactive in its production of protein-digesting enzymes. You may also notice allergies as a result. You need to follow the programme as indicated, and add selenium and strong vitamin B complex.

As a final indicator of possible important nutrients, in which you may be lacking answer the following questions with responses of 'always', 'sometimes' or 'seldom'.
- Do you get backaches?
- Do you feel depressed?
- Are you constipated?

- Do you have pain in your arms, hands, feet or legs?
- Do you find yourself forgetting recent events?
- Do you get cramp at night?
- Do you get out of breath easily?
- Is your skin noticeably wrinkling, or getting coarse?
- Have you indications of varicose veins?

Always means more than once a week. *Sometimes* is more than twice a month, and *seldom* is less than twice a month. You score three for an always, and two for a sometimes, and one for a seldom.

If your score is greater than ten this indicates a tendency to deterioration of general function, and early ageing. The overall programme should help considerably in the reversal of these trends. If you are not already supplementing the following, as a result of the previous questions, then add these to your programme. They are designed to counteract the effects of ageing, as expressed by the sort of symptoms listed above. Most are anti-oxidants, which will protect your body against what are called 'free radicals', which can cause damage to the circulatory and other systems of the body:

Vitamin C; emulsified vitamin A; vitamin E; selenium; strong B complex; l—cysteine (one gram); l—carnitine (one gram); and one gram of glutathione (these last three are amino acids; or amino acid groups, which are safe and protective of vital aspects of the body, in times of stress and exposure to undesirable toxic elements). Also add manganese, calcium and magnesium (all as orotates). Powerful antioxidant, and therefore anti-ageing, enzymes are now known to be useful when supplemented. These are available in a form called OxyPlex from BioCare, who are listed on page 118.

We have now explored a wide range of possible minor health problems which can be clear indicators of a need for nutrient alterations, and/or supplementation. Having

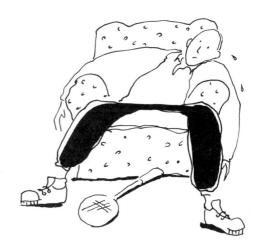

progressed from the point where your diet was over-burdened with undesirable factors, which I hope you have now relegated to the past, and having identified your biochemical and metabolic needs and begun to meet them nutritionally, this last stage is designed to fill any possible gaps that we might have missed. It is in your long term interest to incorporate these suggestions into your now well established programme of nutritional reform; exercise and visualization. In three to six months you should go through this questionnaire again and revise your nutrient supplementation accordingly. It is quite likely that you will be able to cut out most of the additional supplements by then. In order to understand correctly just what you should, and should not, be taking in the way of supplements, I will go through a few of the more obvious pitfalls relating to the selection of these. First, however, consult the list of supplements and relate the number of times these were indicated to each, so as to determine your suggested daily intake.

Supplements

When you determine your required intake, based on the number of times the supplement has been indicated by your answers to the questions, take into account whether that particular supplement has already been suggested in the earlier chapters relating to your metabolic type or endocrine pattern.

If it has, then you must not add the quantities given below it, but include such an indication in assessing your daily quantity. You may have been advised, because of your adrenal gland questionnaire for example, to take vitamin B complex. You may also have answered one question in this last section which indicates that you require vitamin B complex. Opposite you will see that if you have answered 'yes' twice or more to a question which gives such an indication, you should take two vitamin B complex tablets daily. But as you are already taking one, because of the adrenal dysfunction, you only add one extra to take a daily total of two. This would still be the case even if you had four indications for its use.

In other words, the amount given opposite in the right hand column is the *maximum* of any nutrient supplement that I am going to ask you to take, no matter how often in the book it is indicated as necessary. Many people do require greater quantities of certain nutrients, but we are not going into the realms of mega-vitamin therapy in this book. We will stick to what is both safe and effective. Now add up your 'yes' answers in the previous section of this chapter and consult the list opposite.

If copper is taken supplementally it should be at a different time from zinc, and for no longer than six months before complete reassessment is carried out. Taking zinc and copper at the same meal can result in neither being adequately absorbed.

These nutrients are not medicines. They are concentrated foods and should be taken with, or after, meals, unless otherwise indicated. There is every reason to believe that it is all but impossible to meet all nutrient requirements from food alone, once the body is in a chronic state of deficiency. Many current surveys indicate that the majority of people in Western society are deficient in one or more of these nutrient factors. The suggestions above are based upon many years of research, and upon your individualized response to particular questions and tests.

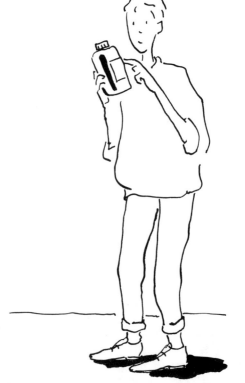

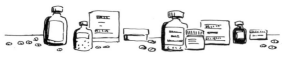

Supplement quantities

Supplement	One Yes	Two or more Yes
Vitamin A (emulsified or water miscible)	10,000iu	20,000iu
Beta-carotene	2,000iu	4,000iu
Vitamin B_1 (thiamin)	10mg	20mg
Vitamin B_2 (Riboflavin)	20mg	40mg
Vitamin B_3 (Niacin)	50mg	100mg
Vitamin B_5 (calcium pantothenate)	100mg	500mg
Vitamin B_6 (pyridoxine)	25mg	100mg
Vitamin B_{12} (cyanocobalamine)	50mcg	200mcg
Vitamin B complex (strong)	1 tablet	2 tablets
Vitamin C	1g	2g
Vitamin E	200iu	400iu
Vitamin F (essential fatty acids)	500mg	1000mg
Calcium (as orotate)	500mg	1000mg
Magnesium (as orotate)	250mg	500mg
Manganese (as orotate)	50mg	100mg
Chromium (as orotate)	10mg	20mg
Copper (as orotate)	10mg	10mg
Iron (as orotate)	50mg	50mg
Zinc (as orotate)	100mg	200mg
Dolomite tablets (calcium and magnesium)	3	4
Brewer's yeast tablets	9	12
Iodine (in the form of kelp)	1g	2g
Selenium	50mcg	100mcg
Tyrosine (amino acid)	200mg	400mg
l-Cysteine (amino acid)	1g	3g
l-Carnitine (amino acid)	1g	3g
Glutathione (amino acid compound)	1g	3g
Inositol	250mg	500mg
PABA	500mg	1000mg
Lecithin	1000mg	2000mg
Bioflavinoids	500mg	1000mg
Alfalfa	500mg	1000mg
Thymus extract (glandular substance)	300mg	400mg
Adrenal extract (glandular substance)	200g	400g
Liver concentrate	300mg	600mg
Thyroid extract (glandular substance)	300mg	600mg
Oxyplex Antioxidant Enzymes	3 capsules	6 capsules

Obtaining your supplements

If you are seeking pure and natural supplements of a type that your body can readily absorb and utilize, then it is vital that you take note of the advice contained in this section. There is little point in purchasing supplements which are going to pass through your body unabsorbed. The term 'bioavailability' is used to indicate that a substance is easily absorbed.

In the case, for example, of the fat soluble vitamins, such as vitamins A and E, there are forms which are much more easily digested and incorporated into your system than others. These are known as 'water miscible', or 'emulsified' forms of the vitamins. They are available if you ask. In most cases your local health store will obtain them, even if they are not readily available on the shelf.

The same applies to the minerals that are indicated (calcium, manganese, zinc, etc.) You will note that I have stressed as ideal the 'orotate' form. This simply means that the mineral has been chelated with a natural substance (a protein) called orotic acid, to increase its bioavailability, and also to aid the transportation of the mineral once inside your body. There are other forms of chelation which are excellent and, if the orotates are difficult to obtain, then at least ensure that all minerals taken are 'chelated'. It will state this clearly on the bottle or package.

With vitamin B complex you will note that I have used the word 'strong' in connection with this tablet. There are many formulas available constituting, more or less, what the total B complex ought to contain. If you are going to derive the maximum benefit from taking a B complex, then it should have as a formula nothing less than the following quantities for the listed contents: vitamin B_1 (thiamin) 50 mg; vitamin B_2 (riboflavin) 50 mg; vitamin B_{12} 50 mcg; choline 50 mg; inositol 50 mg; biotin 50 mcg; folic acid 400 mcg; PABA 25 mg. Ideally, this formula should also contain some vitamin C. You should be able to find such a formula in your local health store.

When selecting a vitamin C it is advisable to look for one that contains bioflavinoids. This will be clearly stated on the label. You should look for a calcium ascorbate, rather than a sodium ascorbate, when reading the label.

As to whether a 'natural' source is more desirable than a synthetic one, it is clear that, ideally, natural is better in terms of biological activity. It is also clear that, in the case of most vitamins, it is not a possibility to provide totally natural supplements, owing to a combination of economics and logistics. In some cases the cost would simply be prohibitive, and in others the size of the natural product would make it necessary to eat a

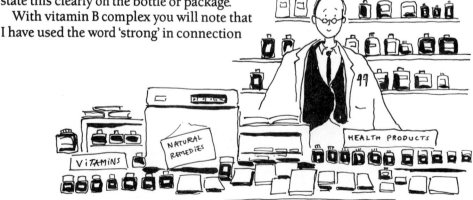

huge amount of a substance in order to obtain what is available in a small tablet via the synthetic source.

In certain cases, say vitamin E, it is known that the natural form, which is readily available, is superior in its biological action to synthetic forms. Look at the label, and ensure that what is in the package is *d*-alpha tocopherol and not *dl*-alpha tocopherol (the synthetic form). In most other nutrients there is a tendency to mix synthetic and natural ingredients (such as adding rose hip or acerola to vitamin C) and this may increase the cost enormously. It is not certain that the advantages are worth such a cost.

In some cases it is possible to go to a raw material for general supplementation. Inositol, for example is obtainable in large quantities from wheatgerm and lecithin. If these are playing a part in your diet, supplementation of inositol itself may be unnecessary if indicated, simply take the raw material source.

Iodine is obtainable from kelp, and vitamin A is readily available from carrots. The best source of the essential fatty acid linoleic acid is Evening Primrose oil. Be sure that this is what you are buying by checking the label carefully.

On page 118 there is a list of suppliers of those supplements listed who will be able to help if you are unable to obtain supplies at your local health store.

Supplement summary

If you have found that there are a number of indications for supplementation, as a result of your answers, then you will also recognize that your current state of health is not what it ought to be. You may not be ill enough, in your estimation, to require medical attention. Indeed, you may not see your minor afflictions as warranting any attention at all, since most people you know are in the same, or worse, condition.

There are people who could go through the lists of questions and emerge at the other end of the book, *with no indications for any supplementation at all*. They would be unusual in this day and age, but they would represent the ideal state of health to which we all aspire. They would be able to say that they honestly feel tip-top all the time; sleep well, have no discomforts, aches or pains; no skin or hair problems; no lack of energy; and that they simply do not know what illness means.

In order to achieve an approximation of the ideal state, you need to reform your lifestyle, diet, exercise pattern, etc. By combining this with positive mental imagery and, above all, by formulating this whole programme around indicators which you yourself have provided, we have arrived at a point where you can put all this acquired knowledge together, and begin to work towards your ultimate goal of health, well-being, and the ideal weight for you.

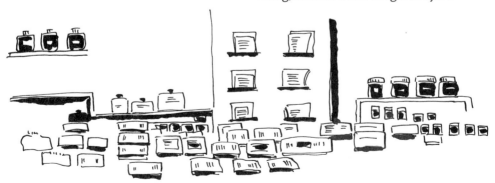

If you are really put off by the supplements listed, I would urge you to give it a try, for three months at least, and six months ideally. Then re-check the whole list of questions and tests and see for yourself just how much you have improved. Compare your answers, and remember just how you felt at the outset. If you wish to apply the programme in a truncated form, then you will certainly derive some benefits for you will, at least, be supplying nutrition according to your metabolic needs. You will, however, lose out on achieving the level of well-being that is possible.

If economic factors mitigate against you following the full programme then I would suggest a modified formula of supplements which would include the following: brewer's yeast (as a source of B vitamins, chromium and selenium); wheatgerm (as a source of B vitamins and vitamin E); kelp (as a source of minerals and iodine); garlic capsules (as a source of sulphur-rich cleansing elements) and vitamin C. At the very least add these to your overall programme in order to support your nutrient levels for the next six months. This is not suggested as a means of escaping the undoubted bother of swallowing a lot of tablets, but as an alternative if you really cannot afford the expense of the whole supplement programme. *Quantities*: brewer's yeast, 2 tablespoons (or 9 tablets); garlic capsules, 3; vitamin C 1g; wheatgerm, 1 tablespoon; kelp, 1g.

Suppliers

The best sources of the supplements listed are reputable, nationally known, suppliers and manufacturers. Some supplements are made in the UK, others are imported. If your local health store cannot meet your needs, as defined above, then contact one of the firms listed below. (These are in alphabetical order rather than in any order of preference.)

Cantassium Co., 225 Putney Bridge Road, London SW15.
Manufacture all minerals in orotate form; glandular substances (such as adrenal), emulsified vitamin A, amino acids, and all other nutrients.

G. and G. Food Supplies, 175 London Road, East Grinstead, Sussex. RH19 1YY. Also import high potency acidophilus powder.

Green Farm Nutritional Supplements Centre, Green Farm, Burwash Common, E. Sussex, TN19 7LX. Import and supply amino acids, glandulars, vitamins and minerals (in chelated forms).

Nature's Best, 1 Lamberts Road, Tunbridge Wells, Kent TN2 3EQ. Import and supply amino acids, glandulars, vitamins and minerals (in chelated forms).

Biocare, 20-24 High Street, Solihull, West Midlands.
Supply high potency enzyme products including Oxyplex.

Putting it all together

In the course of this book you should have discovered a few interesting new facts about yourself. You are the possessor of a particular metabolic type, and it is also possible that you are experiencing the over—or underfunction of certain key hormonal activities. This can be seen as the broad framework from which certain deductions can be made as to your best way of eating. Within that framework we have used a series of questions to uncover particular requirements which you may have in your unique biochemical make-up.

Once we ascertained these, then the whole picture took shape. By using the indicators, together with the information we have (the framework described above) we have arrived at a unique formula which will be suited to your metabolic type, and to your particular needs within that type.

To recap, we have tried to eliminate those things which are 'bad' for everyone from a health and weight viewpoint. We have then established just what physical and metabolic type you are, so that we know broadly what pattern of diet you should be following. All this while we are edging you towards a pattern of exercise, the amount of which will be determined by your own body, because you will use indicators from your physiological response to tell you when you are doing enough.

We have also, introduced certain nutrient supplements, *if they are indicated by particular signs and tests*. The identification of these indicators will show us specific nutritional requirements which are unique to you. Then it was time to begin a pattern of guided imagery. This quite simply means that we will use the power of imagination to

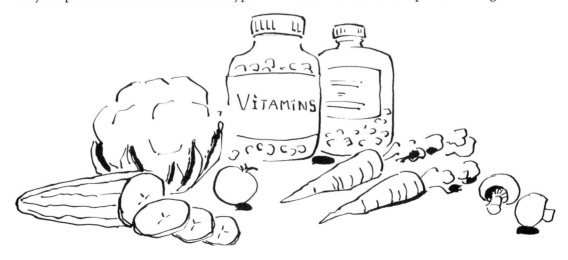

help bring you into touch with aspects of your body, and your attitudes to food, eating, weight, etc., of which you are probably totally unaware.

Finally, to round off this exciting journey towards health and ideal weight, we will discuss some new and revolutionary discoveries relating to appetite and hunger, and little 'tricks' we can play on our appetite control mechanism when bad habits reappear or, if under stress, we are tempted to eat incorrectly (see page 125).

This knowledge will enable us to convince our 'satiety' centre in the brain that it has had enough to eat when we are tempted to overeat.

By combining together, in one programme, all these aspects of health and ideal weight promoting factors, I believe you will have the knowledge which can transform your life, immeasurably improve your health and probably lengthen your life, or at least improve the quality of it.

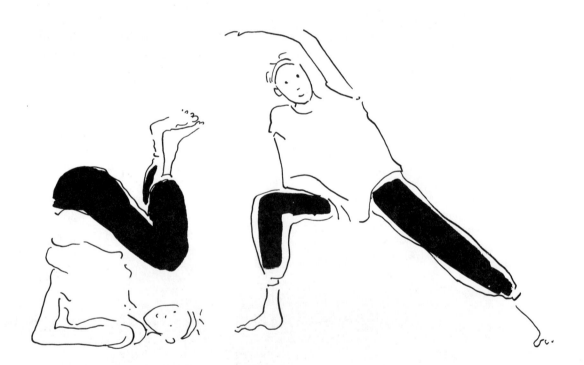

Using the programme

Take it one step at a time. It is important to do things in their proper sequence, since the whole point of the endeavour is to lead you towards a state of health, and this cannot be done without gradual changes which involve mind and body and the combining of the various elements of the programme.

It should be clear to you that no 'system' of dietary change that fails to take into account that you are a unique biochemical and metabolic entity, can possibly hope to do more than have short term effects. We are seeking long-term, revolutionary and evolutionary changes, not flash-in-the-pan results, which are meaningless when seen in the context of a lifetime.

Losing weight is not high on my list of priorities for you. You might lose a lot, but only if you really need to. Remember, our first and most dedicated aim is to achieve a stage of health in which your weight will, as a normal consequence of your condition, be at its optimum. This might well be, in your particular case, a few pounds over, or under, whatever some mythical ideal says it should be. I want you to forget such unscientific and meaningless nonsense and concentrate on making the very most of the wonderful machine with which nature has blessed you.

If there is a secret to this whole programme, and in fact there are many such secrets added together, the main one is this central discovery of our unique physical (diet and exercise) and mental/emotional individuality.

Once we are aware that we are different, and that we must work within the dictates of the individual requirements set for us by nature, we have the marvellous opportunity of achieving health, and with it a rare happiness, contentment, and sense of achievement.

We will have actually met our physiological needs, perhaps for the first time in our lives, and the rewards will flow from that. The ability to use ourselves in an unconstrained manner, with a certainty that our body will respond with the energy and precision that we ask of it, allows life to have a new meaning. This should be your aim. The degree to which you apply yourself will, to a very large extent, determine how well you succeed. The knowledge that you have done it for yourself is the final blessing, for it crowns the achievement and adds to your inner confidence and direction.

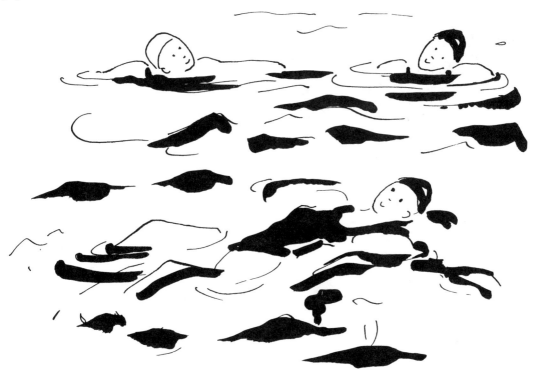

Weight loss

If your reason for reading this book was a desire to lose weight, then there is a need to discuss certain aspects of this problem. You may have found that you have identified your particular type as being more of a draught horse than a racehorse, or more of a bulldog than a whippet. It must be obvious to you that no amount of nutritional or exercise variation is ever going to turn a bulldog into a whippet-shaped dog—it cannot be done. What *can* be done is to make that bulldog as trim and fit as is possible.

This knowledge may not make you happy, but it is a realistic appraisal of the situation. On the other hand, you may be a bulldog or draught horse type, but still be carrying too much weight. If this is so, then be assured that the application of the pattern we have so laboriously covered together will take care of the surplus, and trim you down to your normal and desirable weight.

If you have a long history of being overweight, and have repeatedly tried one diet or another, then you will by now realize that it is not of the slightest use to do the same thing all over again. The only way in which you are going to achieve your goal is applying the basic principles that we have explained in this book, and begin to change your life. As you alter your nutritional and exercise pattern towards what you have found for yourself to be your ideal pattern, you will find that your body will slowly but surely change, and weight will come off. It should not come tumbling off, as this is not desirable.

If you are 20lb (9 kilos) or more above the indicated weight for your height, then a loss of between a half and one pound (250-500g) weekly, over a period of six months, should allow you to approximate your target weight. If you do follow all the advice in the book, regarding both diet and exercise as well as the visualization programme, this should be achieved. And you should be able to maintain your new weight, since your inbuilt defence system, which has foiled previous attempts to slim, will not be alerted into trying to prevent the change in weight.

If you try crash diets you will only achieve heartache, as the weight lost will more than be replaced. The only way to a correct weight loss pattern is via a health promoting pattern which takes into account your individual needs.

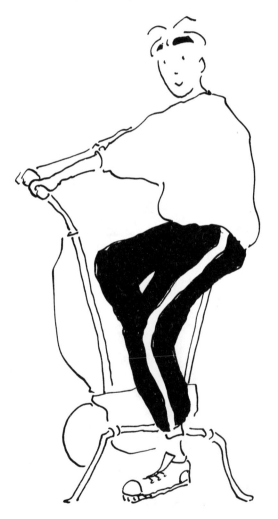

Eating habits

If 'bingeing' and uncontrollable urges to eat are a factor in your past history of dieting, then we should consider aspects of this problem. It is true that we may intellectually realize that a particular action is undesirable, and yet still go ahead and do it. One reason for this is that, if we once react to a situation in a particular manner, even if it is undesirable, we will tend to react in a similar way at each subsequent exposure to that situation.

If, in the face of unhappiness or loneliness, or any other identifiable stress factor, you have been in the habit of turning to food for solace and comfort, then knowing that this is exactly what you should not do is not going to stop you from doing it again. Because you have once reacted in that way you are more likely to do so again, and your intellectual realization of the folly of the act will not stop the urge from expressing itself. It is as though an action seems right on an emotional level, even though logically you know it is unwise.

The way to begin to break this habit is to realize the mechanisms that are at work. If you know that, given a stress situation of any sort, you might be tempted to 'binge' then do so *but in a different way.*

First:
- ensure that the worst of the possible 'tasty toxins' are not easily available. Don't have chocolates, cream buns, cakes, etc., in the house. If they are not there you will not be tempted to eat them.

Next:
- replace them with high-fibre, very chewy substitutes. You might ensure a supply in the house, at all times, of such foods as raw carrots, apples and sugarless wholegrain biscuits. Eat as much of this sort of food, as you wish, if you cannot control your desire to eat. But first try a bit of deception.

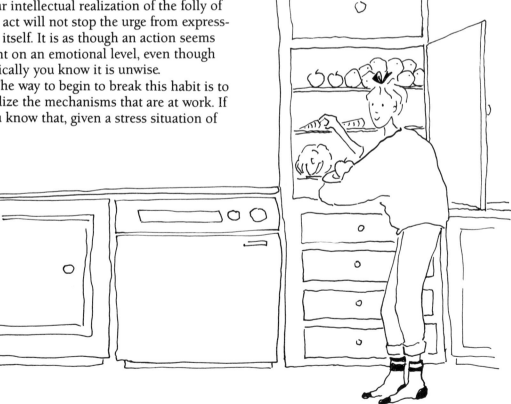

I have explained that because, in the past, you have reacted in a certain way to stress, it feels comfortable to you emotionally, even though you know you shouldn't do it (the guilt adds stress, and makes you even more likely to surrender to the urge). If you can begin to substitute a different reaction then, after a bit of repetition, this will become 'comfortable', and seem the correct thing to do.

This 'something else', can be as varied as going for a walk, or doing something physically active (cleaning the windows, or digging the garden); or quite the opposite—lie down on the floor and tell yourself that if the urge to eat is just as strong after 15 minutes of relaxation and visualization, then you will give yourself permission to binge (but on the high-fibre, chewy foods). One or other of these substitute actions should work for you.

The idea of giving yourself permission to do a thing is of importance. You can learn to see yourself as both a parent and a child. It is the child who wants instant satisfaction, and it is the adult who says, 'all right, but first do this.' By giving the 'adult' part of you the chance to exercise some control over the 'child' in you, you can delay the desire for instant gratification. This, in itself, is very possibly enough to break the habit pattern to which you have previously given way.

You can practise this little delaying action in many ways. Any time that you are about to do something, however trivial, you can say to yourself, 'Yes, but only after I have counted to 30.' This teaches you that it is possible to exercise discipline and control and still, in the end, have the opportunity to do what you wanted to do. It also gives enough time for you to change your mind, or forget all about what it was that you were going to do.

If, despite the delaying tactics, or the vigorous alternative (walking or digging, for example), there is still the feeling of wanting to 'binge', then do so, but on wholefoods. By providing yourself with food that requires a good deal of chewing, and which produces a feeling of fullness and satisfaction far more swiftly, and for far less calories, you will do much less harm than if you were pushing large amounts of pappy, high-carbohydrate junk, into yourself.

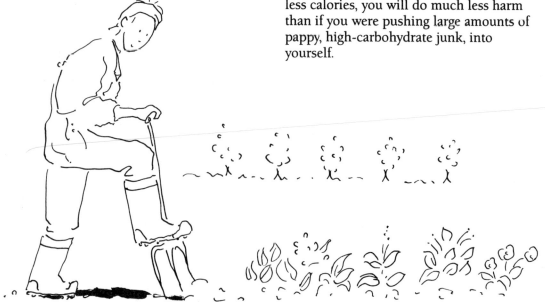

Safe tricks to confuse your appetite

There are a few more devious little tricks that you can attempt in trying to fool your 'child' self. If, at the time you first feel an urge to binge, you take certain amino acids, you may well completely fool the appetite centre in your brain into believing that you have already eaten. It will also make the selection of the food on which you binge more desirable, by reducing your desire for sugary foods. Ensure that you have available a bottle of l-phenylalanine. Before you do any of the things described above take 500 to 1000 mg of this amino acid. Then continue as outlined. Caution regarding phenylalanine should be exercised if you have high blood-pressure, or are taking drugs known as monoamineoxidases (MAO for short).

If sugar craving has been a real problem in your condition the general pattern which has been outlined in the previous chapters should take care of this. You can, however, help this particular problem by taking, on a daily basis, the amino acid l-glutamine. This is a remarkable 'brain food' as well as being helpful in cases of cravings for sugar and alcohol. One gram daily is usually adequate, but some people need more (it's perfectly safe) and trial and error should help you find the level at which your craving disappears.

If excessive appetite in general is a problem for you then, by eating a small snack (say one wholemeal biscuit) of a carbohydrate nature, and at the same time taking a supplement of 300 and 500 mg l-tryptophan about half an hour before your normal meal time, you will induce a situation in which, whether you want to or not, you will be more likely to choose 'safe foods' (as far as calories are concerned) than otherwise. Caution is suggested for any woman who might be pregnant, or about to become pregnant, in taking large doses of tryptophan since, although it is perfectly safe for the adult individual, it might induce birth defects (this as been observed in hamsters, not humans, but the precaution is worth noting). The only other effect that you might notice with tryptophan is a pleasant drowsiness, and a reduction in any feelings of depression.

These tricks are not suggested as long term measures, but as aids to help you through the initial stages, until you begin to see results from the combined programme.

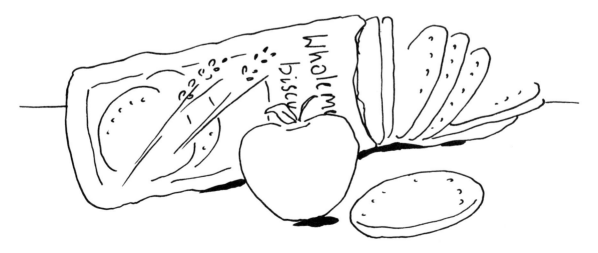

Good luck

You now have all the information you need and you must take up the challenge and go for your goals. The level of health that lies waiting for you is the reward. There could be no greater blessing than to achieve that goal.

Index

adrenal dominant individual, 55
adrenal function, 101
  overactive, 103
  underactive, 48, 101
adrenal metabolism questionnaire, 54
adrenal type, the 67, 69
  exercise for, 69
  menu for, 68, 70
  supplements for, 69, 70
adrenalin (epinephrine), 22
amino acids, 74

Bieler, Dr Henrym 51, 61
BioCare, 118
bingeing, 123-129
blood-pressure test, adrenal, 48
breathing, rhythmic, 43, 90, 91
brown fat, 28

calorie counting, 14
cancer, 22
Candida infection, 70
Cantassium Co., 118
carob, 24
chewing, benefits of, 34
cholesterol, 27
confirmation tests, 58
coronary disease, 22
culinary herbs, 20

diabetes, 22
dietary pattern, basic, 31-33

eating, 34

exercise, necessity of, 37
  toning, 86-89
exercises, stretching, 38-42, 79, 81
  advanced, 82-83

fat cells, 26
fats, 26-28
fitness index, 49-50, 87
flour, refined, 25, 29
food additives, 19, 21
Food Is Your Best Medicine, 51
fructose, 22

G. and G. Supplies, 122
glucose, 22
Green Farm Nutritional Supplements, 118
guided imagery, 93-95

honey, pure, 24
hypoglycaemia, 22

individuality, 11
insurance companies, weight charts used by, 14

Kelley, Dr William, 51, 58

'mixed' type, the, 55
  diet for, 70
  supplements for, 70

Nature's Best, 118
nervous system, 45
nutrient supplements, 114-115
  natural, 116
  necessity of, 113
  suppliers of, 118
nutrients, 60, 114
  in oratate form, 116
nutritional questionnaire, 108-113

obesity, 22, 26
One Answer To Cancer, 51

pituitary dominant individuals, 56
pituitary metabolism questionnaire, 53
pituitary type, the, 64-65, 71
  exercise for, 66
  menu for, 64, 70
  supplements for, 66, 70
programme, results of, 13

relaxation, 43-45, 90

saccharine, 24
salt, 19-20, 29
salt substitute (potassium chloride), 19
sucrose, 22
sugar, 22-24, 29

temperature test, 47

thyroid dominant individual, 55
thyroid function, normal 47
  overactive, 47, 99
  underactive, 47, 100
thyroid metabolism
  questionnaire, 52
thyroid type, the 61, 71
  exercise for, 63
  menu for, 62, 70
  supplements for, 63, 70
tooth decay, 22, 24

visualization, 93-95

walking, benefits of, 86
weight, ideal, 9, 11, 13
  optimum, 13
  problems, 71-72
weight-controlling system, 14